# Disability Rights and Wrongs

Over the past thirty years, the field of disability studies has emerged from the political activism of disabled people. In this challenging re-evaluation, leading disability academic and activist Tom Shakespeare now argues that social model theory has reached a dead end.

Drawing on a critical realist perspective, Shakespeare promotes a pluralist, engaged and nuanced approach to disability. Rather than rejecting research in medical sociology, bioethics and social care, disability studies needs to re-engage with the fundamental questions of what disability is, and how the lives of disabled people can be improved. Topics discussed include:

- dichotomies – the dangerous polarisations of medical model versus social model, impairment versus disability and disabled people versus non-disabled people
- identity – the drawbacks of the disability movement's emphasis on identity politics
- bioethics in disability – choices at the beginning and end of life, and in the field of genetic and stem cell therapies
- care and social relationships – questions of intimacy, friendship and the role of non-disabled people.

This stimulating and accessible book challenges British disability studies orthodoxies, and promotes a fresh research agenda. It will be required reading for researchers and students in disability studies, medical sociology and social care, and will have applications for professionals, policy-makers and activists.

**Tom Shakespeare** has taught and researched sociology at the Universities of Cambridge, Sunderland, Leeds and Newcastle. He has written and broadcast extensively about disability and genetics, and his co-authored books include *The Sexual Politics of Disability*, *Exploring Disability* and *Genetic Politics*.

# Disability Rights and Wrongs

## Tom Shakespeare

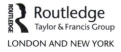
Routledge
Taylor & Francis Group

LONDON AND NEW YORK

First published 2006
by Routledge
2 Park Square, Milton Park, Abingdon, Oxon, OX14 4RN

Simultaneously published in the USA and Canada
by Routledge
270 Madison Ave, New York, NY 10016

Reprinted 2006, 2007 (three times)

*Routledge is an imprint of the Taylor & Francis Group, an informa business*

© 2006 Tom Shakespeare

Typeset in Times New Roman by
Keystroke, Jacaranda Lodge, Wolverhampton
Printed and bound in Great Britain by
TJ International, Padstow, Cornwall

All rights reserved. No part of this book may be reprinted or
reproduced or utilised in any form or by any electronic,
mechanical, or other means, now known or hereafter invented,
including photocopying and recording, or in any information
storage or retrieval system, without permission in writing from
the publishers.

*British Library Cataloguing in Publication Data*
A catalogue record for this book is available from the British Library

*Library of Congress Cataloging in Publication Data*
A catalog record for this book has been requested.

ISBN10: 0–415–34718–1 (hbk)
ISBN10: 0–415–34719–x (pbk)
ISBN10: 0–203–64009–8 (ebk)

ISBN13: 978–0–415–34718–1 (hbk)
ISBN13: 978–0–415–34719–8 (pbk)
ISBN13: 978–0–203–64009–8 (ebk)

Dedicated to the memory of Mairian, Paul and Peter

# Contents

# Chapter 1

# Introduction

Since 2000, the disability movement in Britain appears to have stagnated. Despite important and progressive changes in wider society, the politics of disability seem to have run out of steam. Partly, this may be a consequence of the success of the disability rights agenda. Following the adoption of the disability discrimination legislation for which the disability movement had campaigned for so long, there has been a lack of clarity about future priorities. Meanwhile, mainstream disability organisations and agencies have taken on some of the central tenets of the disability rights philosophy. And there is also a generational effect, as many of the activists who emerged in the 1970s and 1980s have retired or died. Yet I believe that this lack of progress may also indicate the failure of radical approaches based on the social model of disability, which have sometimes become inward-looking and sectarian.

Over the same period, I and others have been writing and talking about the need for a new approach to understanding disability, which enables research and practice to progress, forms new alliances, and advances an agenda of disability equality. This work has been controversial. However, I suspect that there is support, agreement and interest in new approaches from many quarters, and therefore I have tried to consolidate my ideas and work in different fields in the current volume. At the outset, my intention was to reprint various existing papers. Because there were overlaps, ommissions, and aspects which I felt it necessary to revise, I have taken the opportunity of writing a substantially new work. The resulting book brings together about a decade's worth of thinking and talking about disability, bioethics and care. It represents my attempt to establish a balanced, rational and coherent analysis of disability, which will be of value to practitioners, researchers, and disabled people themselves. I have particularly tried to ensure that issues concerning people with learning difficulties are not ignored (Chappell, 1998).

The book draws on my experience of being a disabled person, and the son, father, husband and friend of disabled people. It has been influenced by my personal experience of disabled people's organisations and other voluntary organisations. It draws on qualitative research I have conducted over the past decade, as well as the wealth of research on disability within disability studies and medical sociology. Discussions with philosophers and professionals have also been very valuable to me in shaping my ideas. The resulting book is not a straightforward work of academic social science. It draws on other disciplines – particularly philosophy – and has an emphasis on policy, practice and politics. The target audience includes disabled people and those who work with them, as well as academics and policy-makers. I have tried to write clearly and accessibly, with a view to helping non-academics think deeper about questions which matter in their lives, as well as contributing to a reinvigorated and empirically based disability studies.

## Outline of the book

In the first part of the book, I reject the strong social model approach to disability and attempt to construct an alternative which neither reduces disability to an individual medical problem, nor neglects the predicament of bodily limitation and difference. In recent years, I have come to the conclusion that the British social model version of disability studies has reached a dead end, having taken a wrong turn back in the 1970s, when the Union of Physically Impaired Against Segregation (UPIAS) social model conception became the dominant UK understanding of disability. It appears to me that disability scholars in other countries do not have the same problem, because they have adopted a less dogmatic version of the social approach to disability. Here, I try to show that it is possible to have a radical and progressive disability politics without relying on a strong social model formulation of disability.

The first chapter looks at what I call the family of social-contextual approaches to disability. Here I have tried to show that the social model is not the only progressive way of understanding disability. By looking at accounts prior to the 1976 'Fundamental Principles' document produced by the UPIAS, and by looking at disability theory in different countries, I demonstrate that there are different options for de-medicalising disability and promoting social change to enable and include people with impairments. The second chapter focuses directly on the British social model of disability. First, I demonstrate the political dangers of treating the social model as a litmus test. Then I explore different problems with the model itself: the neglect of impairment, the dichotomy between impairment and disability, and the faith placed in barrier removal. I acknowledge that the slipperiness of the social model makes any criticisms hard to sustain, but believe I have demonstrated in this chapter that the model lacks firm foundations. In the third chapter, I begin to construct an alternative account of disability, which is based on an interactional or relational understanding. Disability results from the interplay of individual and contextual factors. In other words, people are disabled by society *and* by their bodies. This approach bridges the political gulf between the medical and social models of disability, and can be related to the World Health Organization's International Classification of Function, Disability and Participation. In the fourth chapter, I explore the complex issues in disability identity, questioning whether the disability rights movement can represent the diversity of disabled people, and suggesting that identity politics can be as much an obstacle as a solution.

In the second part of the book, I explore several bioethical questions relevant to disability: genetic screening at the beginning of life; the endeavour to cure impairment; assisted suicide and other end of life issues. Here again I provide an alternative account to the ideologies which have dominated disability rights thinking. For example, I argue that it is important both to prevent impairment and to support the rights of disabled people, and that these two responses to the disability challenge are not incompatible. My ethical position is influenced by engagement with analytic philosophy, although I believe that a virtue ethics approach is a necessary correlative to the utilitarian arguments which sometimes dominate thinking in bioethics (Gardiner, 2003). Attention to emotions and situations can balance the emphasis on individual autonomy and rationality. As Dan Callahan argues, 'Rationality is important, but it is never enough. The worst possible mistake on the part of philosophers, all too common, is to think that good ethics comes down to good arguments' (Callahan, 2003: 288).

Everyday life is more complex and nuanced than philosophers sometimes allow for, and to this extent I agree with Zygmunt Bauman's call for a postmodern ethics:

> Human reality is messy and ambiguous – and so modern decisions, unlike abstract ethical principles, are ambivalent.
>
> (Bauman, 1993: 32)

I believe that more engagement between disability studies and bioethics would be beneficial for both parties. (Kuczewski, 2001)

In the third part of the book, I broaden my focus to reflect on disability and social relationships, looking at topics such as charity, care, friendship and independent living. I argue that rights alone are not sufficient to promote the wellbeing of disabled people, and that charity – defined broadly as love and solidarity – must also play an important part. The first versions of some of these arguments were first outlined in *Help* (Shakespeare, 2000). It may become clear in this final section that my anxieties about individualism and rights are part of a broader personal philosophy which, albeit incoherently expressed, has affinities with virtue ethics (Macintyre, 1999) and the feminist ethics of care (Tronto, 1993).

Needless to say, the present book does not provide a comprehensive account of disability. It excludes important areas – employment, education, housing, transport – where I have done little or no work. However, I hope that my approach has relevance to these other areas of disabled people's lives. The book also neglects important topics – cultural representation, childhood – where I have done work, but which could not be included due to problems of space and coherence. Moreover, while I have rooted my analysis in empirical evidence wherever possible, I am conscious that there is a pressing need for new qualitiative and quantitative data in disability studies, which makes me feel slightly embarrassed to be offering yet another volume of theory.

## My academic journey

Like all researchers, my personal background and experience of disability have influenced my work in disability studies, and so it seems appropriate to include a brief description of my personal journey. I have the genetic condition achondroplasia, the commonest form of restricted growth or dwarfism. I inherited it from my father, William Shakespeare (1927–96), who was a general practitioner. Ignorance and prejudice was a stronger factor in his life than it was in mine, and he had to overcome negative attitudes in order to achieve professional status. He brought me up to consider myself the equal of non-disabled people, and to have high aspirations. Widely admired as a doctor and as a disabled role-model, his example has also influenced my attitudes to medicine.

I had the advantage of a privileged background: I attended private school and Cambridge University, where I ended up studying social and political science. As a radical student, I supported liberation movements such as feminism, anti-racism and lesbian and gay rights. Studying sociology, and active in left politics, it was easy for me to make analogies with my personal experience of disability. I helped write a disability access guide to Cambridge University and became active in the National Union of Students, where I met other left-wing disability activists including Martin Pagel and Stuart Bracking. After working for two years, I returned to college to do an M.Phil. and then a Ph.D. For my M.Phil. dissertation in 1989–90, I wrote about the politics of disability, using ideas drawn from Marxism, from feminism and from Mary Douglas' concept of anomaly. At this stage I had not encountered the social model, although I was convinced that a social-contextual approach to disability was necessary.

Wanting to expand the dissertation into a book, I registered for a Ph.D. Almost immediately, I encountered Michael Oliver's *The Politics of Disablement* (1990) and Jenny Morris' *Pride Against Prejudice* (1991). Morris' account fitted better with my developing understanding of disability, because of my growing interest in cultural imagery and prejudice. As someone with a very visible impairment, being stared at and made fun of has always been my main encounter with oppression, and this has influenced my approach. It's interesting to note that Mike Oliver and other wheelchair users have often stressed environmental barriers in their work, whereas Susan Wendell (1996), who has ME/CFS (Myalgic Encephalomyelitis/ Chronic Fatigue Syndrome), discusses her personal experience of pain and fatigue. Perhaps disabled scholars often emphasize the dimension of disability which they most directly experience.

My doctoral thesis was an account of different ways of conceptualising disability. While the thesis was never published in its entirety, individual chapters became articles (Shakespeare 1993, 1994) and my paper 'What is a disabled person?' (1999b) summarises the overall approach. Because I had come to the social model only after I had started to think of disability as a political issue, I was always a critical friend: one of my earliest publications was a supportive response to Liz Crow's famous *Coalition* article about impairment (Crow, 1992; Shakespeare, 1992).

Aspects of my biography and interests partly explain my subsequent research choices. Becoming a parent in 1988, which included passing my impairment onto my children, deepened my interest in genetics and eugenics (Shakespeare, 1995a). As a member of Regard (the national network of disabled lesbians, gays and bisexual people) and as I explored my own sexuality, I became interested in the neglected issue of disability and sexuality. When Dominic Davis suggested we collaborate professionally, I worked with him and Kath Gillespie-Sells to produce *The Sexual Politics of Disability* (1996), one of the first UK accounts of disabled sexuality. As the parent of disabled children, it was natural to investigate disability in childhood. The responses our team gathered from young disabled people helped further challenge my reliance on a social model framework for understanding disability (Priestley *et al.*, 1999). So did my experience of serious back problems in 1997: for the first time in my life, my impairment caused me serious pain and restrictions, which gave a renewed impetus to my attempts to give space to impairment within my account of disability.

My back problems made the prospect of commuting from Tyneside to Leeds unacceptable, and so I took up a new job, developing the Policy, Ethics and Life Sciences Research Institute, a collaboration between the University of Newcastle, University of Durham and the new Life Science Centre. This also corresponded with my growing interest in genetics and bioethics (Shakespeare, 1995a, 1998, 1999a). I was unprepared for the vicious reaction from several members of the disability movement nationally and locally to my new role researching the social and ethical aspects of genetics.

This episode marked the beginning of a breakdown of my relationship with the mainstream of the UK disabled people's movement. My work became increasingly critical of the social model of disability, and many activists saw this and my genetics work as a betrayal. Although I had founded two disability organisations on Tyneside, I never felt able as an independent academic to allow the disability movement to dictate my research approach or agenda, when so often I found activist approaches inadequate or contradictory. Listening to doctors and to parents challenged my own prejudices, and forced me to engage with difficult questions. Engaging with philosophers exposed the limitations of my arguments, and of the social model tradition in general. I came to the conclusion that UK disability studies was too reliant on political rhetoric and ideology, and that many core assumptions needed to be tested and even rethought. This led to the paper 'The social model of disability: an outdated ideology?' which I wrote with Nick Watson (Shakespeare and Watson, 2001a). The first section of the current book builds on that paper and my subsequent thinking.

I cannot claim to have been consistent in my writings on disability. At one time I was a critical friend of the social model, defending it against external attack (Shakespeare and Watson, 1997): I am now among those who argue that it should be abandoned. My initial radical rejection of genetic screening (Shakespeare, 1995a) has now been replaced by a more nuanced understanding, as evidenced by chapter 6 in this volume. My work has always represented my current best thinking on the issue in question, and my fundamental commitment to the liberation of disabled people has been unchanging. All my work has aimed to promote better understandings of the complexity of disability, and better outcomes for disabled people. I have tried to be honest and open, and to be as critical of my own work as I have been of that of others. I believe that it is important for disability studies to be pluralist, and to recognise that there are diverse views among disabled people, and different responses to the complex questions raised by disability. Foreclosing debate, or promoting a single and often simplistic answer, does not seem helpful.

Although I have often disagreed with my disability studies colleagues on particular points, I have greatly appreciated the advice, inspiration, dialogue and affection I have found among the disability studies community throughout the world. In particular, I want to acknowledge the input and feedback of many colleagues, including Bill Albert, Jerome Bickenbach, Mark Erickson, Lars Grue, Kristjana Kristiansen, Helen Meekosha, Jackie Leach Scully, Carol Thomas, Rannveig Traustadóttir, Bryan Vernon, Fiona Williams and in particular Nick Watson. Among the doctors who have challenged and inspired me, I thank in particular John Burn, Joanna Cox and Michael Wright. Among the many philosophers who have provided patient critical feedback or offered suggestions, I thank Richard Ashcroft, John Harris, Richard Hull, Michael Parker, Janet Radcliffe Richards, and in particular Simo Vehmas and Simon Woods. At home, Caroline Bowditch and Ivy Broadhead have given me both emotional and intellectual support. Needless to say, none of the foregoing are responsible for my errors and ommissions.

I first corresponded with Paul Abberley at the beginning of my postgraduate studies, and admired his theoretical contributions to British disability research. Mairian Scott-Hill (formerly known as Mairian Corker) was a highly original and charismatic theorist with whom I was privileged to work on the 'Life as a Disabled Child' project and an edited collection of disability theory. I met Peter Bryan as an activist in Newcastle disability politics. An organic intellectual of the highest calibre, most of his extensive writings remain unpublished. Paul, Mairian and Peter would have argued with many of my claims in this book, and their criticisms would have been worth listening to very carefully. Each could be a warm and generous companion, and their premature deaths are a major loss to the UK disability community. This book is dedicated to their memory.

# Part I

# Conceptualising disability

# Chapter 2

# The family of social approaches

## Introduction

*social model*

This book is my attempt to offer a way beyond the impasse of British disability studies. While I value the achievements which have been won through the close alliance of disability politics and disability research, I believe that the weaknesses of the British approach now outweigh the benefits. Translation of ideas and ideologies from activism to academia has not been accompanied by a sufficient process of self-criticism, testing and empirical verification. The social model of disability which has successfully inspired generations of activists has largely failed to produce good empirical research, because it relies on an overly narrow and flawed conception of disability.

It is vital to state that in rejecting the social model of disability, I am not rejecting a political approach to disability. Many activists and writers in the UK appear to believe that the British social model is the only appropriate or effective analysis or definition of disability. It almost seems as if there is an acceptance that without the social model there can be no political progress and no social movement of disabled people. If I believed that this was the case, it would be very much more difficult for me to suggest that the social model should be rejected or replaced. For those who hold this belief, it is understandable that they might view my work, and that of other critics inside and outside the disability community, as unacceptable.

In this chapter, I will demonstrate that the social model is not the only progressive account of disability. Instead, I will claim that the British social model is just one of a family of social-contextual approaches to disability. All of these approaches reject an individualist understanding of disability, and to different extents locate the disabled person in a broader context. To varying degrees, each of these approaches shares a basic political commitment to improving the lives of disabled people, by promoting social inclusion and removing the barriers which oppress disabled people. If the social model is one member of a broader family of progressive approaches, it might be helpful to investigate how British activists have come to see it as unique and indispensable. During the 1960s, 1970s and 1980s there were different, competing social-contextual approaches to disability even within the British disability movement, yet I trace below the process by which the social model became dominant over other rival approaches.

It is also important to understand the way in which the social model has been counterposed to the 'medical model'. To activists, the power of the latter has made the need for the former more urgent. Since its outset, most British disability studies have relied on binary distinctions (though see Priestley, 1998 for an exception). One of the claims of this book is that many of these distinctions are misleading and dangerous. The impairment/disability distinction is perhaps the primary dichotomy, but the distinction between the social model and the medical model runs it a close second. Just as Marxist social theory distinguished itself from bourgeois social theory, so British disability studies has distinguished the right way – defined in terms of a social model perspective – from the wrong way represented by the medical model. Whereas many contributors to UK disability debates take the idea of the medical model for granted, it might be better to deconstruct the concept.

British disability studies has been slow and reluctant to take on research from disability researchers in other parts of the world. Because most non-British disability studies research has not been based on the impairment/disability distinction and has not adopted the strong social model version of the social-contextual approach, it has been conveniently ignored or rejected as inadequate or mistaken. Yet to view non-British research in this way is to be too fixated with terminology – as if using the phrase 'people with disabilities' rather than the preferred 'disabled people' invalidated an entire research agenda. For example, *Disability is not Measles* was an important and radical North American collection of research about disability. Reviewing the book, Colin Barnes (1995) acknowledges its many strengths, before complaining that it uses the World Health Organization International Classification of Impairments, Disabilities and Handicaps (ICIDH) definitions not British social model definitions, as if this invalidated the volume. In 1998, Barnes took the same approach to Susan Wendell's important American analysis, *The Rejected Body* (1996). In 1999, he repeated the same critique in the context of another US book, Simi Linton's *Claiming Disability* (1998). British disability studies thinking has sometimes been guilty of marginalising or ignoring the contribution of other social-contextual approaches to understanding disability and researching disabled people's experiences, particularly those from other countries.

## Establishing the year zero

By looking back at the origins of the British social model, it is possible to trace how an important and unarguable insight – that many of the problems which disabled people face are generated by social arrangements, rather than by their own physical limitations – evolved into a rigid ideology claiming that disability was everything to do with social barriers, and nothing to do with individual impairment. Examining the history carefully shows how in Britain, one particular form of the social-contextual approach to disability – the social model – triumphed over other, less extreme, versions of disability politics. The legend is of a polar switch: the social model replaced the medical model, thanks to the pioneering activists of UPIAS and the academics who followed them. The truth is that there was, and always has been, a plurality of social approaches, the most extreme version of which triumphed and has become the orthodoxy of the British disability movement and of British disability studies. Over at least four decades, and in many different countries, social scientists and disability campaigners have regarded disability as bound up with social-context, and have drawn attention to the disadvantage, social exclusion and even oppression experienced by many disabled people. But only the British social model redefined disability as oppression.

The Union of Physically Impaired Against Segregation (UPIAS) was one of a number of disabled people's organisations which emerged in the 1970s. The Disablement Income Group (DIG) had formed in 1966, and campaigned on a platform of improved benefits for disabled people. However, DIG had not developed a critique of residential institutions, nor a broad based campaign for disabled people to have control over their own lives. Frustration with DIG drove both the formation of the Marxist-inspired UPIAS, as well as that of the Disability Alliance, a more reformist group which offered an alternative solution to the social problems of disabled people.

UPIAS originated when Paul Hunt, a resident of the Le Court Cheshire home, wrote a letter to the *Guardian* newspaper which was published on 20 September 1972, calling for the formation of a consumer group to represent those living in institutions. Hunt had spent his childhood, and much of his adult life, in residential institutions. He had actively researched independent living, inclusive education and welfare benefits, through contacts with the USA and Nordic countries. In 1966, he had edited *Stigma*, a collection of essays by disabled people reflecting on the prejudice and exclusion they experienced. Another key player in UPIAS was Vic Finkelstein, a spinal cord injured psychologist. In 1968, Finkelstein, subjected to a banning order by the South African apartheid regime for his civil rights activism, came to Britain as a refugee. He was able to make the connection between the liberation struggles of black South Africans and the situation of disabled people. Paul Hunt, Vic Finkelstein and others created UPIAS (Finkelstein, 2001). For their first couple of years, the network seems to have concentrated on discussion and debate, in the attempt to develop a political ideology of disability.

According to their resulting policy statement (adopted December 1974), the aim of UPIAS was to replace segregated facilities with opportunities for people with impairments to participate fully in society, to live independently, to undertake productive work and to have full control over their own lives. The policy statement defined disabled people as an oppressed group and highlighted barriers:

> We find ourselves isolated and excluded by such things as flights of steps, inadequate public and personal transport, unsuitable housing, rigid work routines in factories and offices, and a lack of up-to-date aids and equipment.
> (UPIAS Aims paragraph 1)

However, the policy statement did not contain a definition of disability as social barriers or as oppression. The terms 'physically impaired people' and 'disabled people' were used interchangeably, and in one place there is a reference to 'physical disability'. The statement called for alliances with other groups – such as the 'mentally handicapped' and 'mentally ill' – and with non-disabled allies. However, only people with physical impairments were eligible to become full members of UPIAS, and there was clearly a fear of being taken over by non-disabled people.

The first surviving statement of what was to become the social model of disability came in the publication *Fundamental Principles of Disability*, which reported on discussions in November 1975 between UPIAS and the Disability Alliance. Founded in 1974, the Disability Alliance was a cross-impairment grouping which sought to promote a comprehensive income scheme. Chaired by the academic Peter Townsend, it sought to bring together a coalition of disability groups and disabled individuals, with non-disabled academics and experts. The Alliance agreed with UPIAS that disability was a social problem, but argued that financial problems were fundamental to the isolation and segregation of disabled people. UPIAS demanded a more comprehensive response, not just a continuation of the previous DIG focus on incomes. Unlike the Alliance, which was a coalition of existing disability groups, UPIAS explicitly set out to create a mass grass-roots organisation of disabled people.

The 'Fundamental Principles' which formed the starting point of the discussions between the two organisations were written by Paul Hunt, and at the outset defined disability as follows:

> [D]isability is a situation, caused by social conditions, which requires for its elimination, (a) that no one aspect such as incomes, mobility or institutions is treated in isolation, (b) that disabled people should, with the advice and help of others, assume control over their lives, and (c) that professionals, experts and others who seek to help must be committed to promoting such control by disabled people.
>
> (UPIAS, 1976: 3)

The Disability Alliance felt able to subscribe to this view. During the discussion itself, recorded on the third page of the document, UPIAS elaborated their position on disability:

> In our view, it is society which disables physically impaired people. Disability is something imposed on top of our impairments, by the way we are unnecessarily isolated and excluded from full participation in society. Disabled people are therefore an oppressed group in society.
>
> (UPIAS, 1976: 3)

This is a more precise development of Paul Hunt's fundamental principle, which explicitly distinguishes impairment from disability in a way which the 1974 Policy Statement does not do. The statement continues as follows:

To understand this it is necessary to grasp the distinction between the physical impairment and the social situation, called 'disability', of people with such impairment. Thus we define impairment as lacking all or part of a limb, or having a defective limb, organism or mechanism of the body and disability as the disadvantage or restriction of activity caused by a contemporary social organisation which takes little or no account of people who have physical impairments and thus excludes them from participation in the mainstream of social activities.

(quoted in Oliver, 1996: 22)

This further formalises the impairment/disability distinction. UPIAS clearly had a developing position: it is clear that between the first Policy Statement and the Fundamental Principles document, their position had strengthened. Even within the Fundamental Principles document, it is possible to see the social model definition of disability as social exclusion becoming more specific and definitive. When the sociologist Michael Oliver became involved with social model theory in the early 1980s, the impairment/disability distinction was further reinforced at the core of the disability rights ideology.

My claim in this reading of the origins of the UK disability movement is that the source of the current fruitless and frustrating debate about the social model of disability lies in the increasingly ideological definition of disability which developed from the initial insights of Paul Hunt and his colleagues about the social factors in disabled people's experience. A good idea became ossified and exaggerated into a set of crude dichotomies which were ultimately misleading.

In retrospect, UPIAS has been celebrated as the inspiration for the British disability movement, and as the pioneers of the social model. It was certainly the intellectual and political heart of the movement. But distance and mythology risk obscuring its limitations. It never grew into a mass movement. It was dominated by wheelchair users, perhaps because many had previously been able-bodied, and had been involved with other political movements (Finkelstein, 2001: 4). Some activists remember it as being sexist (Campbell and Oliver, 1996: 52), and as dominated by a typically masculine form of politics, which was hard, ideological and combative (Campbell and Oliver, 1996: 67). It seems to have operated Leninist democratic centralism, meaning that after discussion and agreement, dissent from the party line was not tolerated: individuals who disagreed either left the network, or were expelled.

The UPIAS/Oliver social model was not, and has never been, the only social-contextual approach to understanding the disability experience. The 1970s and 1980s were decades when disabled people were emerging from the shadows, partly due to increased access to education. Many initiatives flourished in different areas of the country: arts groups such as Graeae; housing initiatives; advice projects; women's groups and consciousness raising groups. For example, an important alternative approach to disability politics was offered by the Liberation Network of People with Disabilities. The Liberation Network, like UPIAS, were clear that disability was a form of social oppression. Their draft Liberation Policy, published in 1981, argued that while the basis of social divisions in society was economic, these divisions were sustained by psychological beliefs in inherent superiority or inferiority. The Liberation Network accepted that people with disabilities, unlike other groups, suffered inherent problems because of their disabilities. Their strategy for liberation included: developing connections with other disabled people and creating an inclusive disability community for mutual support; exploring social conditioning and positive self-awareness; the abolition of all segregation; seeking control over media representation; working out a just economic policy; encouraging the formation of groups of people with disabilities.

Significantly, the Liberation Network policy statement stressed that they welcomed the comments and contributions of others. It appears that theirs was a more fluid politics, which both involved women as leaders, and reflected a less workerist and more feminist style. There is a clear contrast between the Liberation Network's open style, stressing individual transformation and mutual support, modelled on feminism and personal growth, and the more coherent and disciplined approach of UPIAS, modelled on labour movement politics. As in other revolutionary periods, it was the more organised, coherent and ideological faction which won out, and consequently the UPIAS style and ideology became dominant within the British Council of Organisations of Disabled People (BCODP), founded in 1981.

After the formation of Disabled People's International (DPI) in 1981, Finkelstein and the other BCODP delegates argued, at the Singapore Congress, for the DPI constitution to be based on social model definitions (Dreidger, 1989). The definitions of disability adopted in 1982 marked a further development of the original UPIAS social model. Impairment was defined as 'the functional limitation within the individual caused by physical, mental or sensory impairment' and disability as 'the loss or limitation of opportunities to take part in the normal life of the community due to physical and social barriers' (Disabled People's International, 1982). These definitions show the incoherence which had entered into the debate. First, the definition of impairment is circular: impairment is functional limitation caused by impairment. Second, the definition of disability contains no mention of impairment. In other words, disability now covers any exclusions due to physical or social barriers, which would include members of many other socially excluded groups: women, poor people, ethnic minorities and others.

The legend of the origins of the British disability movement creates a year zero – 1976, the publication of the UPIAS *Fundamental Principles of Disability* – and a strict dichotomy – medical model versus social model. Anything prior to 1976 can be discounted. Any account of disability which is not based on the distinction between impairment and disability becomes 'medical model' and hence unacceptable. Ironically, leading disability studies academics have repeatedly urged more junior scholars not to forget the past and to cite the pioneering writings of the 1970s and 1980s, rather than 'reinventing the wheel'. Yet the advocates of the social model have themselves often been guilty of ignoring any pioneering research conducted outside the UPIAS tradition.

## Deconstructing the medical model

The original policy statement of the Union of Physically Impaired Against Segregation, adopted on 3 December 1974 and amended on 9 July 1976, does not use the terms medical model or social model. It was Michael Oliver who in 1983 conceptualised the binary distinction between what he called the individual and the social models. Oliver had not been a UPIAS member, and had been introduced to their ideological contribution in his work for the Open University course team which produced the 1981 collection, *Handicap in a Social World*. In his 1996 account of this great leap forward, he conceded 'there is no such thing as the medical model of disability, there is instead, an individual model of disability of which medicalisation is one significant component' (Oliver, 1996: 31).

Again, in his seminal 1990 text, *The Politics of Disablement*, Oliver rarely uses the terms medical model and social model. Instead, he distinguishes 'personal tragedy theory' from 'social oppression theory' (Oliver, 1990: 1), arguing that 'an adequate social theory of disability as social restriction must reject the categories based on medical or social scientific construction and divorced from the direct experience of disabled people' (Oliver, 1990: xiii).

But despite the fact that the medical model/social model distinction is not a central element in the founding formulations, it has come to be a defining characteristic of disability studies in the United Kingdom. The extent to which an academic or an organisation or a policy uses the terminology of the social model or the medical model has become a litmus test of their worth. In particular, disability equality training has advocated replacing 'medical model' with 'social model' responses to disability.

What, then, is the medical model? In a general sense, many disability studies authors have rejected medicalisation, defined as the dominance of medical approaches and of medical experts. Thus 'Our Union rejects entirely any idea of medical or other experts having the right to tell us how we should live, or withholding information from us, or taking decisions behind our backs'. Note that this laudable sentiment in the 1974/1976 UPIAS policy statement is preceded by explicit acknowledgement of the need for medical care and allied therapies.

But disability studies is hardly pioneering in rejecting the dominance of medical professionals or medical definitions. As we have seen, Oliver prefers to use the term 'personal tragedy theory' or 'the individual model', by which he means more than the dominance of doctors or of diagnoses. For him, this means an approach which regards the disability problem as inhering in the individual, and stemming from functional limitations or psychological losses (Oliver, 1996: 32), as opposed to a social model approach which sees disability as arising from restrictions and disabled people as an oppressed group.

No authors have ever explicitly affiliated themselves to this medical model or individual model perspective. But many disability activists, disability equality trainers and disability studies authors have found a convenient symbol of the medical model, in the form of the International Classification of Impairments,

Disabilities and Handicaps (ICIDH). For example, international activist Rachel Hurst has called the ICIDH 'This official, international, underpinning of the medical model of disability' (Hurst, 2000: 1083).

Very frequently, the ICIDH tripartite definition is contrasted with the social model dichotomy. The ICIDH defines impairment as 'any loss or abnormality of psychological, physiological or anatomical structure or function' (World Health Organization, 1980: 27). Impairment is defined as deviation from a biomedical norm, and includes functional limitation. Disability is then defined as any restriction or lack, resulting from impairment, of ability to perform an activity in the manner or within the range considered normal. Finally, handicap is 'a disadvantage for a given individual, resulting from an impairment or disability, that limits or prevents the fulfilment of a role that is normal (depending on age, sex, and social and cultural factors) for that individual' (World Health Organization, 1980: 14).

But when the ICIDH was developed for the World Health Organization by Phillip Wood, Michael Bury and Elizabeth Badley their intention was to move away from medical definitions and diagnoses, and to create a framework which would make space for the social experiences of disabled people (Bury, 1997: 138). Michael Bury states that:

> Our aim, it will be remembered, was to challenge the medical model and assumptions about disablement. Most importantly, our aim was to bring handicap onto the healthcare agenda. That is, we were pressing for greater recognition of (what came to be called) social exclusion in response to disablement.
>
> (Bury, 2000: 1074)

He further argues that the ICIDH stressed the consequences of health-related phenomena, with the intention of increasing recognition of the social disadvantage experienced by many disabled people. Bury claims that, far from being an oppressive medical model, the ICIDH has been beneficial to the lives of disabled people. Elsewhere, despite his resistance to the 'over-socialised social model', he has clearly stated that disability is a relational concept (Bury, 1997: 119).

While Bury may be right to see the ICIDH as a step forward from previous narrowly medical approaches, the ICIDH remains deficient, in failing to capture the way in which environments, facilities and policies make a huge difference to the extent to which an individual with impairment is able to function and fulfil their role (Edwards, 2005). As Michailakis has argued, 'The distinctive feature of the individual-centred approach to handicap is the disregard for the constraining force of values and social structures' (Michailakis, 1997: 22).

Jerome Bickenbach et al. (1999) argue that the ICIDH does recognize the role of social environmental factors, but concede that,

> although identified as a classification of 'circumstances in which disabled people are likely to find themselves', there is never any reference in the

handicap classification to features of the social world that create those circumstances. It is a classification of limitations of people's abilities.

(Bickenbach *et al.*, 1999: 1175)

While handicap was intended to be a socialised concept, it remains dependent on impairment and disability, rather than being based on the relationship between an individual and their context. It is impossible to use the ICIDH to record how environmental changes can lead to changes in an individual's functional abilities. It is clear why the fledgling disability movement in the UK opposed the ICIDH definition. However, despite these deficiencies, the ICIDH has benefits, and can be used accurately to describe some dimensions of disabled people's experiences. There are many examples of progressive research projects or policy statements which have relied on ICIDH definitions. In some ways, and for some uses, it is preferable to the vagueness of the UPIAS and DPI definitions. It therefore seems unfair to equate the ICIDH with the 'medical model'.

Looking elsewhere for 'medical model' accounts, it is not difficult to find sociological accounts of disability from the 1970s and 1980s which take an individualist approach to explaining disabled people's problems. For example, Eda Topliss published *Social Responses to Handicap* in 1982. Although non-disabled herself, her sister had a progressive neurological disorder, so she had some personal experience of disability. Her account is a compassionate study of the disadvantages faced by disabled people. However, she does not attend to the contribution of environments, policies and provision in creating the disability problem. For her, handicap is intrinsic to the individual, arising from the loss of function caused by impairment. In a competitive economic environment, in which independence is highly valued, she argues that disadvantage will inevitably be the consequence of having an impairment.

Clearly, it was even common for disabled people themselves to take an individualist approach to understanding disability in the post-war period. For example, Tremblay *et al.* (2005) explore the post-war history of wheelchair use in Canada, showing how an individual approach to disability predominated. When wheelchair users encountered problems getting around, they did not intepret these environmental barriers as the problem:

Central to the life experiences of these civilian pioneers was the belief that individuals needed to adapt to existing environments and that wheelchairs were obstacles to participation, not steps and curbs.

(Tremblay *et al.* 2005: 112)

Disabled people became proficient in doing wheelies up and down curbs, rather than calling for curb cuts: only in the late 1960s and early 1970s did civil rights protestors call for barrier removal.

What these different accounts and approaches confirm is that the traditional view of disability was an individualised one. In particular, there was a dangerous tendency to medicalise disability. Yet, it seems to me dangerous to conclude that the distinction between medical model approaches and social model approaches is robust. For example, there were many sociologists and psychologists in Britain and America who were drawing attention to environmental barriers and social relationships during the 1970s and 1980s (Safilios-Rothschild, 1970; Albrecht, 1976; Carver and Rodda, 1978; Laura, 1980; Crewe and Zola, 1983; Marinelli and Dell Orto, 1984; Stone, 1985). To take just one example, the same year as the UPIAS Fundamental Principles, Constantina Safilios-Rothschild had argued:

> The institutionalisation of barrier-free cities, buildings, roads and inside and outside environments would make life easier for and many more options accessible to not only the disabled but also pregnant women, infants, persons pushing baby carriages or pulling grocery carts, old people, and individuals with broken legs.
>
> (Safilios-Rothschild, 1976: 50)

as well as suggesting 'The time may be ripe for the disabled to generate a social movement patterned after the at least partially successful examples of the Black Movement and the Women's Movement' (Safilios-Rothschild, 1976: 43).

Moreover, during the 1960s and 1970s many authors criticised 'medical models', medicalisation and professionalism (Illich, 1977; Goffman, 1968a; Goffman, 1968b; Szasz, 1974; Zola, 1977). Many of these approaches share the spirit of social model approaches, but none of them make the distinction between impairment and disability which defines the social model approach. Goffman in particular has been criticised by British disability studies writers (Barnes, 1998b).

In the decades since UPIAS, the concepts of the medical model and social model have been polarised and reified. The medical model may have been identified with the ICIDH, but it means much more than a simple set of definitions: it has become a proxy for all that it is wrong with traditional attitudes to disability. It stands for research and practice developed by non-disabled people, without the participation of disabled people. It stands for the dominance of professionals. It stands for the idea that disabled people are defined by their physical or intellectual deficits. It stands for medicalisation. The concept of the medical model has become a powerful symbol, but when closely analysed, it is nothing but a straw person.

In his powerful demolition of social constructionism, Ian Hacking (2000: 17) suggests that the term 'essentialism' is not purely descriptive in debates about social theory. It is used as a slur word, in order to put down the opposition: no one, not even the most biological of determinists, stands up and says 'I am essentialist about race'. The term 'medical model' works in similar ways: it is impossible to find anyone who actively espouses the concept. The opposition of 'medical model' to 'social model' is more about symbolism than actual content. 'Medical model' is not a coherent or useful concept. As Kelly and Field have argued, in the context of medical sociology, it is actually very hard to find this medical model in practice. Few practitioners and no textbooks of any repute subscribe to uni-directional causal models and invariably interventions are seen in medical practice as contingent and multi-factorial.

(Kelly and Field, 1994: 35)

I believe it is necessary to rehabilitate pre-social model and non-British disability research, in order to rescue the important insights and findings of other scholars from the dustbin marked 'medical model'. This deconstruction process might lead to the conclusion that the British invention of the social model was not quite the watershed in disability research that many accounts suggest. Exploration shows that many others were coming to similar conclusions about the disabling world, prior to Oliver and parallel to UPIAS.

## Forerunners of the social-contextual approach

Until someone has done systematic historical research, it is only possible to unearth tantalising clues to pre-1975 social-contextual approaches. For example, Irving Zola cites research by William Frey which demonstrates that, as far back as 1958, the American Medical Association was differentiating between impairment and disability:

the former was generally regarded as a medical judgement call whereas the latter was defined as an administrative issue relating to 'the interaction between the impairment and a host of non-medical factors such as age, sex, educational level, economic and social environment.'

(Zola, 1994: 53)

While broadly individualist, Beatrice Wright's 1960 study of the psychological aspects of disability discusses the interaction of people with disabilities with others, the importance of other people's attitudes, the social environment, the way that context can prevent disabilities becoming handicaps, the minority group status of people with disabilities and many of the relational and psycho-emotional features of disability. David Wasserman cites Jacobus tenBroek's 1966 argument that disabled people's rights not only required changes to the built environment, but also imposed duties on non-disabled people in public places; 'the refusal to make these changes denied the disabled their right to live in the world as much as the exclusion of blacks and women from public facilities' (Wasserman, 2001: 240).

In Sweden, Hedlund (2000) shows how biological and social approaches to disability have been contested at least since the 1960s. In Canada, an early statement about the barriers to disabled people's participation dates from 1967 (Mann, 1967). After 1970, however, references to environments, attitudes and other social restrictions become common in disability and social policy literature in Britain and America. This was presumably influenced by the first stirrings of disability activism, following the example of civil rights and feminism, as well as the academic dominance of labelling theory and other conflict theories in sociology.

Sociological research would be expected to contextualise individual phenomena, including disability. Michael Bury (2000) claims that medical sociology has always recognised social setting in which disability is experienced. For example, the British medical sociologist Mildred Blaxter took an interactionist approach to disability in *The Meaning of Disability* (1976), exploring the 'career' of disabled people discharged from hospital. Her study showed the lack of congruence between medical labels, administrative categories and the definitions adopted by the disabled person themselves and their families. Blaxter saw impairment as forming a continuum, not a polar opposite to normality, and regards labels as often arbitrary. She used the concept of stigma, rather than the more political concept of discrimination, but often talks about similar constraints imposed on the disabled people she interviewed:

> fettered and constrained not only by their social environment, but also within the two major systems of society within which their lives were structured: the system of medical care and the administrative system of welfare, employment and social security.
>
> (Blaxter, 1976: 246)

Other medical sociologists came to similar conclusions. For example, David Locker's 1983 study argued that the social consequences and social-context of impairment were as much, or more than, a problem as the impairment itself:

> The immediate context is handicapping where it presents barriers which must be negotiated, consuming reserves of time, money and energy in the process, or where the effort is such that the person decides not to bother and retreats into an enforced passivity. It is also handicapping to the extent that it leaves the individual with no option but to rely on the help of others.
>
> (Locker, 1983: 90)

For Locker, 'handicap' was dynamic and socially generated:

> The extent to which functional limitations and activity restrictions cause a problem, or are otherwise handicapping, is not only variable historically and culturally but is also somewhat dependent on more immediate contexts: their meaning is not the same across different social and environmental settings.
>
> (Locker, 1983: 5)

Substituting 'disabling' for 'handicapping' in these quotations produces a good fit with social model perspectives.

The collection *Disability in Britain: a manifesto of rights* (Walker and Townsend, 1981) emerged from the Disability Alliance grouping. Yet in their introduction, the editors are clear about the need to challenge traditional approaches to disability: 'In sum, there are environmental and psychological barriers to the integration of people with disabilities, but there are also significant financial, social and economic barriers which are fundamental and inescapable' (Walker and Townsend, 1981: 16). Walker returns to the theme in his conclusion. 'Underlying the deprivation of people with disabilities is a social rather than a physical restriction of access to resources and customarily accepted roles and relationships' (Walker and Townsend, 1981: 186). The collection argues for community living, rather than institutions; uses the language of rights; provides data about the poverty of disabled people; argues for benefits to be provided in cash, rather than kind; and Ann Shearer's chapter even calls for comprehensive anti-discrimination legislation. She comments, 'A law is required which asserts that all people with disabilities have the right to share the opportunities that the rest of the population takes for granted, and the right to the help they may need to make this possible' (Shearer, 1981: 87).

In his own chapter about older disabled people, Townsend challenges a 'loss of faculty' approach, saying, 'The medical model lays emphasis upon precautionary and therapeutic action within medicine and sets great store by medical technology' (Townsend, 1981: 93). He argues instead for a 'social model of disablement' – 'The social model lays emphasis on adjustment both to the physical environment and to the variety of roles which individuals play and the relationships they have and are expected to have, as members of society' (Townsend, 1981: 93). Note that this seems to be one of the earliest uses of the medical model/social model dyad, predating Oliver's 1983 adoption of the terminology, although the two models are defined differently. Another difference is that although Walker concludes the book by calling for leadership by disabled people, not experts and professionals, the *Disability in Britain* collection is dominated by non-disabled academics and writers.

*The Experience of Handicap*, published the following year, was written by David Thomas, a non-disabled lecturer in special education. The references to the work of Vic Finkelstein and to the emerging struggle for civil rights suggest that the author's ideas were influenced by the disability movement. While he retains a WHO terminology, he seems to appreciate the social creation of disability:

> The concept of disadvantage allows us to appreciate that disability should be perceived as a relationship. That impairments can lead to disabilities and handicaps is in part a function of a society which is organized and structured for and on behalf of the dominant able-bodied.
>
> (Thomas, 1982: 11)

Overall, however, his study focuses more on impairment than on social restrictions, with the exception of the attention he pays to negative attitudes. His is a liberal response to emerging activism: 'In arguing that society "manufactures" handicap, we must take care not to overstate the case and imply that the problems of disabled people are other people, or that limitations due to impairments are not real' (Thomas, 1982: 173).

While none of these different accounts uses the exact terminology of the British social model, and in that sense a disability studies critic might label them all 'medical model', the analysis they develop often parallels social model formulations. Disability, for all of these authors, is not simply a matter of biology, nor is it an objective departure from norms. Instead, attention is paid to the meaning, expectations, roles and relationships which operate in society. Nor would it be fair to classify all these approaches as social constructionist, in the sense of defining disability in terms of individual attitudes and cultural values (see Albrecht, 1981). In many accounts, material factors – environments, poverty, discrimination – are also regarded as significant.

## De-institutionalisation and normalisation

A very important source of social-contextual approaches to disability is found in normalisation theory. This important area of work, focusing on de-institutionalisation of people with learning difficulties, has been largely neglected within British disability studies (Stalker *et al.*, 1999). Theories of normalisation were developed in the 1960s and 1970s by non-disabled academics, predominantly in the Nordic countries and the United States. The Nordic approach was based on rights:

> The normalisation principle means making available to all mentally retarded people patterns of life and conditions of everyday living which are as close as possible to the regular circumstances and ways of life of society.
>
> (Nirje, 1980: 33)

However, social role valorisation, Wolf Wolfensburger's approach which became dominant in the US and influential in many other countries, stressed social devaluation (1972), and could be criticised as suggesting that people with learning difficulties should fit in with the mainstream and not associate with one another. More radically, John O'Brien (1987) stressed community presence, mainstream facilities, choice over life, opportunities to develop skills to reach potential, respect and community participation. Wolfensburger (1989) went on to criticise the growth of human service industries, and the way their clients became dependent and devalued. Despite early criticisms from social modellists, more recently there has been signs of a growing mutual interest between social model and normalisation approaches, based on some similarities of values and objectives (Tregaskis, 2004a; Race *et al.*, 2005). The non-participation of disabled people themselves in normalisation research can perhaps be explained by the concentration on people with learning difficulties, whose participation in research remains limited even today, partly because of the nature of intellectual impairment. However, normalisation did foster a changed approach to intellectual impairment, and it was under these auspices that self-advocacy and inclusive research has developed in the 1990s and 2000s.

Other researchers and activists working with people with learning difficulties developed accounts which overlap even closer with the British social model. For example, key to the social model of disability is the inversion of traditional causal explanations: rather than the individual with impairment being the problem, the problem is the failure of systems and environments to include and accommodate that person. This radical move of turning things on their head is also the basis of another approach, the Try Another Way system developed by Marc Gold in the late 1960s. This was a method of conceiving of people with learning difficulties in particular which rejected labelling and deficit models. A key principle was that a lack of learning is more about poor teaching than inability on the part of the learner. Gold and his associates were trying to develop a way of maximising the potential of people then labelled as retarded, based on equality and mutual respect. Their aim was status enhancement and community integration. Although Marc Gold himself died of cancer in 1983, his ideas have continued to be developed and applied by Marc Gold Associates (see www.marcgold.com).

To take another radical example, Robert Bogdan and Douglas Biklen also built on the 1960s interactionist tradition of 'thinking about handicapped people as societally created rather than as a natural or objective condition' when they introduced the concept of 'handicapism' in a 1977 paper in the journal *Social Policy*. They defined 'handicapism' as 'a set of assumptions and practices that promote the differential and unequal treatment of people because of apparent or assumed physical, mental or behavioural differences' (Bogdan and Biklen, 1993: 69). For them, 'handicapism' had three components: prejudice, stereotype and discrimination. Their article goes on to identify many issues which would become central to social model analyses of disability: segregation of children in special schools; prejudicial media imagery; oppressive terminology; lack of physical access; inaccessible information; employment discrimination; institutionalisation; charity; labelling; research based on handicapist assumptions. In conclusion, Bogdan and Biklen state:

> We hope that the handicapism paradigm will enable researchers and practitioners to begin to reassess their assumptions concerning segregated service, differential treatment, the real source of the disability problem, labelling and language patterns, and funding mechanisms tied to labelling . . . While we have not yet explored the full ramifications of handicapism, we have attempted to provide the foundation for conceptualizing the experience of handicaps in a way that will not perpetrate prejudicial notions, but rather will help reveal and eradicate injustice.
>
> (Bogdan and Biklen, 1993: 75)

## The minority group model

Radical or social-contextual North American approaches to disability were not limited to the area of learning difficulties. US disability activism had begun in the

1960s, and led to the development of independent living approaches, most famously in Berkeley. In 1973, activism led to the adoption and implementation of Section 504 of the Federal Rehabilitation Act, which prohibited discrimination in federally funded services (Zola, 1983: 56). The US disability movement has paralleled the UK disability movement in its campaigning, advocacy and independent living work (Anspach, 1979). Yet only recently have US concepts of disability drawn explicitly on the UK social model approach.

While North American theorists and activists have developed a social approach to defining disability, these perspectives have not gone as far in redefining 'disability' as social oppression as the British social model. Instead, the North American approach has mainly developed the notion of people with disabilities as a minority group, within the tradition of US political thought. Minority group writers have argued that prejudice and discrimination against people with disabilities have to be combated through civil rights legislation, which will guarantee individual rights. While the work of Crewe *et al.* (1983), Hahn (1985, 1988), Albrecht (1992), Amundsen (1992), Rioux and Bach (1994), Davis (1995) and Wendell (1996) explores important social, cultural and political dimensions of disability, none have made the firm distinction between (biological) impairment and (social) disability which is the key to the British social model. Susan Wendell, for example, adopted the ICIDH schema for her social constructionist account of disability, and retained the idea that disability is about restriction of activity (Wendell, 1996; Thomas, 1999). Colin Barnes writes:

> [M]ost American and Canadian accounts are impairment specific in that they limit their discussions to 'people with physical disabilities' or the body; 'disability' is both biological condition *and* a social construct, and the terms 'disabled people' and 'people with disabilities' are used interchangeably. As Mike Oliver has repeatedly made clear, this is about far more than simply 'political correctness'. It's about the crucial issue of causality, the role of language, its normalising tendencies and the politicisation of the process of definition.
>
> (Barnes, 1999: 578)

Yet these US minority group approaches are clear about the role of the social environment. Back in 1978, Frank Bowe's study entitled *Handicapping America* discussed six forms of social barrier: architectural, attitudinal, educational, legal, occupational and personal. Harlan Hahn writes about the disadvantage of a person with disability which 'stems from the failure of a structured social environment to adjust to the needs and aspirations of citizens with disabilities rather than from the inability of a disabled individual to adapt to the demands of society' (Hahn, 1986: 128).

More recently, Ron Amundsen (1992) has taken a philosophical approach to rooting disability in environmental restriction, while Martha Russell (2002) and Ruth O'Brien (2001) share the materialist approach of UK social model theorists such as Oliver and Barnes. A US collection such as *The Ragged Edge* (Shaw, 1994) echoes many of the concerns of disabled activists and academics in the UK. While US theorists may not usually define disability in strict social model terms, the overarching orientation is social and cultural, not medical or individualist. A similar situation pertains in Australia, where disabled and non-disabled activists and researchers have developed a vigorous and engaged account of disability, use the 'people with disabilities' terminology, and are bemused and alienated by endless British arguments about the social model (Clear, 2000; Meekosha, 2004; Newell, 1996; Goggin and Newell, 2005).

## The Nordic relational model

The Nordic countries, with their extensive welfare states, have a long history of disability research, mainly oriented around evaluation of services (Gustavsson *et al.*, 2005). The notion of normalisation has been particularly influential. Most disability researchers are non-disabled, and there is not the close connection between disability research and disability activism which has been a feature of American and British disability studies. However, the social-contextual approach to disability has been an aspect of Nordic research.

The use of an umbrella term (*funksjonshemming*) for 'disabled people' originated in the 1960s: while it retained a medical implication, it was more neutral than previous descriptors. However, it became associated with an 'environmental turn': as the 1967 Norwegian White Paper on disability stressed: 'Rather than expecting that disabled people one-sidedly shall adapt to society, we also need to adapt the environment to them' (Stortingsmelding 88, 1966–67).

The policy document also called for an end to segregated services, and a recognition of disability rights. During the 1970s this 'reversed adaptation' grew into a definition of disability which stressed 'mismatch' between the individual and the environment: this led to a gradual downplaying of the medical aspect of disability. The term *funksjonshemming* became equivalent to 'disability' (disabling barrier) rather than 'disabled' (a person descriptor): the term being neutral as to whether the obstacle is in the person or the environment. The notion of environments expanded to include not just physical environment, but also social structures (Tøssebro, 2004). In the Nordic languages, as in many other cultures (Stone, 1997, 1999), the UK distinction between impairment and disability is hard to translate, because there are not separate words which can capture the sense of individual bodily experience and social-contextual experience.

The core features of the Nordic relational approach are, according to Jan Tøssebro:

1   A disability is a mismatch between the individual and the environment. This occurs both because of individual differences, and because the environment is not adapted to accommodate the range of people. A deaf person is thus not disabled in a setting where everyone speaks sign language.

2    A disability is also situational. A person with a visual impairment is not disabled when using the telephone. Whether a specific individual limitation becomes disabling or not is linked to concrete situations.
3    A disability is relative, a continuum rather than a dichotomy. The cut off point in impairment-based disability definitions is to some extent arbitrary.

While this relational understanding of disability is widely adopted in the Nordic countries as a theoretical commitment and political principle, it has arguably not had a major practical effect. There seems to have been a failure to operationalise the relational concept when it comes to welfare provision, which continues to rely on medical diagnoses and legitimation, or to education, which uses psychological labels, or even research, which is often based on defining particular populations of people with disabilities (Tøssebro and Kittelsaa, 2004). Moreover, there is lack of emphasis on oppression and discrimination – possibly because these factors are less evident in the historically generous Nordic welfare states. For these reasons, Nordic disability research could be said to resemble mainstream UK disability research in social policy and medical sociology. However, there are clearly also strong similarities between the UK social model approach and the Nordic relational approach.

## Conclusion

In this chapter I have tried to show the range and complexity of approaches to disability, in order to challenge the disability studies dichotomy between the social and medical models. My claim is not that UPIAS or Finkelstein or Oliver plagiarised the ideas of others, or even that the development of the social model was inspired or influenced by interactionism or medical sociology. In many cases, it was no doubt the activists that influenced the academics. For example, Bogdan and Biklen were well aware of 1970s US disability rights activism, which no doubt influenced their thinking about handicapism. The reason for citing these accounts is to undermine the mythical dichotomy between 'medical model' and 'social model' thinking, and to show that important insights about the social creation of the disability problem would occur to many people, disabled and non-disabled, in the decades following the 1960s wave of grass-roots radicalism and the ensuing liberation movements. Colin Barnes has conceded that progressive approaches to disability can be found outside the British disability studies field. Reviewing the work of Albrecht, Stone (1985), Wolfensburger and others discussed above, he concludes:

> Undoubtedly each of the above represents, to varying degrees, an alternative to conventional individualistic interpretations of disability, yet they each fail to address some of the key structural factors precipitating their application. Indeed, in common with much of the literature on disability, they draw on the work of established academics rather than that produced by disabled people and their organizations.
>
> (Barnes, 1998b: 71)

For Barnes, the work of Finkelstein, Oliver *et al.* has three advantages over what has come to be labelled 'medical model' analysis: first, these authors are disabled themselves, and working in the context of disabled people's organisations; second, they root disability oppression in the context of capitalist developments; third, they distinguish between impairment and disability, concentrating on environmental and social barriers (Barnes, 1998b, 76). Criticising contemporary disability studies writers for failing to give credit to earlier accounts by disabled people, Barnes seems content to ignore the contribution by non-disabled academics and activists outside disability studies, or who do not share the ideological commitments of mainstream social model theory.

My argument in this chapter is that there has been a dangerous political tendency to assume that progressive approaches are impossible in the absence of the social model, or to label any rights-based or humanitarian response as 'social model', regardless of the definitions adopted: in other words, social model comes to stand for 'good research and practice' and medical model comes to stand for 'bad research and practice'. To take just one example of this very common tendency in UK disability studies, Jonathan Coles (2001) has researched the application of the social model to people with learning difficulties. Meeting a progressive human service worker, Gary, who sees people as individuals not diagnostic labels, and promotes their rights, Coles assumes that Gary has to be following the social model. This presents Coles with a paradox, because:

> Gary had not encountered the social model, and yet his practice seemed to be drawing more on the social than the individual or medical models of disability. Perhaps it is now seeping into both training curriculae and the wider culture, or perhaps Gary's social values already included a recognition and respect for all human beings and a commitment to equality, when he came into this service.
>
> (Coles, 2001: 509)

There is only a paradox here if it is assumed that only those who adopt the social model are capable of respecting rights and individuality and promoting inclusion. Yet, as I have shown above, there are many approaches to disability which stress these values and goals. The social model is not unique, nor is practice and policy doomed if it fails to accept social model definitions.

For further evidence of how medical model/social model dichotomies are created and sustained, I turn to Michael Oliver's book *Understanding Disability* (1996: 34) which includes a table listing the differences between the 'individual model' and the 'social model'. In the first column, Oliver lists words such as 'medical-isation', 'adjustment', 'prejudice', 'attitudes', 'care', 'policy'. These are taken to be negative and reactionary terms redolent of the individual or medical model. In the second column, Oliver provides progressive alternatives: 'self-help', 'affir-mation', 'discrimination', 'behaviour', 'rights', 'politics'. In his commentary on this table, Oliver concedes that it should not be taken as representing a set of dichotomies. He comments, 'It should be noted that, like all tables, this one oversimplifies a complex reality and each item should be seen as the polar end of a continuum' (Oliver, 1996: 33), but at the same time he wants to reinforce the importance of the oppositions being drawn – 'Nevertheless, underpinning [the table] is the same fundamental distinction between impairment and disability as defined by UPIAS' (Oliver, 1996: 33).

It seems that Oliver wants to have his cake and eat it too. It is difficult to interpret what is meant by the table at all, which seems difficult to operationalise. Much the same applies to the famous table in his seminal *Politics of Disablement* (1990), which contrasted what he saw as the individualist questions used in the 1988 OPCS Disability Surveys with the social model approach he preferred. For example, instead of asking 'What is wrong with you?' (medical model), Oliver offers 'What is wrong with society?' (social model). While this reversal is stimulating and suggestive, it seems unlikely that Oliver's questions would have produced reliable and valid data, either about the numbers of disabled people, or about the specific natures of disabling barriers.

By showing that the social model is not unique, but is part of a family of social-contextual approaches, I want to make a further and more radical suggestion. Disability studies would be better off without the social model, which has become fatally undermined by its own contradictions and inadequacies. To reject the British social model does not mean returning to the bad old days of medicalisation and individualist approaches before the UPIAS revolution. There are many other, more robust, ways of conceptualising disability, which retain a commitment to equality and justice for disabled people, but do not base the analysis on a mistaken bracketing of bodily difference.

# Chapter 3

# Critiquing the social model

Few new truths have ever won their way against the resistance of established ideas save by being overstated.

Isaiah Berlin, *Vico and Herder* (Berlin, 2000)

## Introduction

The social model of disability has been called 'the big idea' of the disability movement (Hasler, 1993). To many, it appears to be the fundamental political principle which both first initiated and now sustains the disability rights challenge. For these advocates, to abandon the social model would be to abandon the whole edifice of disability rights and disability equality. Yet the social model itself is a very simple and brief statement which turns the traditional definition of disability on its head. As the UPIAS activists argued:

> In our view, it is society which disables physically impaired people. Disability is something imposed on top of our impairments, by the way we are unnecessarily isolated and excluded from full participation in society.
>
> (UPIAS, 1976: 3)

The benefits of the social model approach are that it shifts attention from individuals and their physical or mental deficits to the ways in which society includes or excludes them. The social model is social constructionist or, as Michael Oliver (1990) prefers, social creationist, rather than reductionist or biologically determinist. Rather than essentialising disability, it signals that the experience of disabled people is dependent on social context, and differs in different cultures and at different times. Rather than disability being inescapable, it becomes a product of social arrangements, and can thus be reduced, or possibly even eliminated.

The redefinition of disability in the social model parallels the feminist movement's redefinition of women's experience in the early 1970s. Anne Oakley (1972) and others had distinguished between sex – the biological difference between male and female – and gender, the socio-cultural distinction between men and women, or masculine and feminine. The former was biological and universal, the latter was social, and specific to particular times and places. Thus it could be claimed that sex corresponds to impairment, and gender corresponds to disability. The disability movement was following a well-established path of de-naturalising forms of social oppression, demonstrating that what was thought throughout history to be natural was actually a product of specific social relations and ways of thinking.

The social model was crucial to the British disability movement for two reasons. First, it identified a political strategy: barrier removal. If people with impairments are disabled by society, then the priority is to dismantle these disabling barriers, in order to promote the inclusion of people with impairments. Rather than pursuing a strategy of cure or rehabilitation, it is better to pursue a strategy of social transformation. In particular, if disability could be proven to be the result of discrimination (Barnes, 1991), then campaigners for anti-discrimination legislation saw civil rights – on the model of the Americans with Disabilities Act, and the British Equal Opportunities and Race Relations laws – as the ultimate solution.

The second impact of the social model was on disabled people themselves. Replacing a traditional deficit approach with a social oppression understanding was and remains very liberating for disabled individuals. Suddenly, people were able to understand that it was society which was at fault, not themselves. They didn't need to change: society needed to change. They didn't have to be sorry for themselves: rather, they could be angry. Just as with feminist consciousness raising in the 1970s, or with lesbians and gays 'coming out', so disabled people began to think of themselves in a totally new way, and to become empowered to mobilise for equal citizenship. Rather than a demeaning reliance on charity, disabled activists could now demand their rights.

In academia, the social model opened up new lines of enquiry. Whereas the medical sociology of disability had traditionally investigated issues such as individual adjustment to impairment and explored the consequences of impairment for identity, the social model inspired researchers in the new field of disability studies to turn their attention to topics such as discrimination, the relationship between disability and industrial capitalism, or the varying cultural representations of people with impairment. The social model enabled the focus to be widened from studying individuals to exposing broader social and cultural processes. Disability studies consciously emulated the precedents of Marxism, feminism, lesbian and gay studies and post-colonial studies which had all asked new questions and generated new insights and evidence on the basis of an overt political affiliation with social movements of liberation.

This brief sketch signals how real and how widespread the benefits of the disability rights movement have been in Britain. The Disability Discrimination Act of 1995 and its successors, the removal of barriers to access, the development of independent living and direct payments, have all begun to transform British society. Given that, in Britain, disability rights and disability studies have up to this point been inseparable from the social model concept, then clearly credit has to be paid to the mobilising power and strategic impact of the social model redefinition of disability. Activists created the social model, which inspired new generations of activists, who fought for the structural changes which the social model mandated.

It is impossible to know whether the British disability movement would have moved so far, or so fast, in the absence of the social model. Certainly, disability rights in other countries have progressed just as quickly, and in some cases rather further, in the absence of the strong version of the social model. As I argued above, this suggests that while a social approach to disability may be indispensable, it does not have to take the particular form of the British social model. Indeed, the strength and simplicity of the social model of disability has created as many problems as it has solved.

## The political dangers of the social model of disability

Perhaps only the most powerful counter-claim could have effectively dislodged the deep seated idea that disabled people are defined by their incapacity. So from one extreme – the cultural assumption that disability is equated with dependency, invalidity and tragedy – the disability movement swung to another – the political demand that disability be defined entirely in terms of social oppression, social relations and social barriers. From seeing disability as entirely caused by biological deficits, the radical analysis shifted to seeing disability as nothing whatsoever to do with individual bodies or brains. This unprecedented movement to turn traditional views of disability upside down appears, several decades later, to be one of the bravest and most transformative moves in the history of political thought, because it goes against deep-seated intuitions and appears to defy logic. However, consistently applied, the social model created entailments which generated problems both at the political and the conceptual level. Here are some of the difficulties which arise from the implications of the social model:

1   If disabled people share a common experience of oppression, regardless of impairment – just as black people share a common experience of racism, regardless of ethnic origins – then to organise or analyse on the basis of impairments becomes redundant. Both impairment-specific organisations – whether traditional charities, or modern self-help groups (see for example Hurst, 1995) – and impairment-specific responses become problematic. Michael Oliver argues that 'the social model is incompatible with taking an impairment specific approach to disabled people' (Oliver, 2004: 30). The only exception Oliver concedes is the need for specific services for Deaf people. It should be noted that Finkelstein (2001) differs from Oliver on this point.

2   If disability is about social arrangements, not physical or mental impairments, then attempts to mitigate or cure medical problems may be regarded with intense suspicion. They will appear to be irrelevant or misguided responses to the true problem of disability, and distractions from the work of barrier removal and civil rights.

3    If disability is not to be understood in terms of individual experiences, but as
     the product of structural exclusion, then the number of disabled people no
     longer becomes relevant. The imperative for social change and disability
     provision is to remove environmental and social barriers, rather than to meet
     the special needs of impaired individuals. Thus it is not necessary to survey
     the impaired population, nor to know how many people there are with each
     form of impairment.

     Rejection of single-impairment organisations, of medical interventions, and
of surveys of disabled people were all persistent features of the UK disability
movement in the 1980s and 1990s. This seems to be evidence of how rigid social
model thinking became problematic and counter-intuitive. There appears to be no
intrinsic reason why a single-impairment organisation might not be progressive
and helpful, given that people with different impairments experience specific
issues and problems, both medical and social. Nor is it logical to think that a focus
on social barriers necessitates a neglect of medical intervention. To accept – or
even to prioritise – wider structural change does not necessitate the abandonment
of medical research or clinical interventions. Finally, understanding the number of
disabled people in society would seem to be important for many different areas
of social policy in the real world of budgetary constraints and service planning.
For example, an inclusive school system would need to provide special needs
assistants for disabled pupils, and therefore it would be important to understand
how many people might need those services. Fully including Deaf people would
require provision of sign language interpreters, and therefore it would be necessary
to know how many Deaf people are present in a particular locality in order to
provide enough interpreters (Harris and Bamford, 2001). Surveying any social
category necessitates a potentially arbitrary definition of the population being
counted, and in that sense, an unavoidable circularity results: the numbers found
are an artefact of the definition used (Abberley, 1992). Yet the constructed nature
of the disability category does not mean that there is no point in such surveys,
simply that each survey can only be understood in terms of the purposes for which
it was intended and the definition of a disabled person on which it relies.
     These cases are examples of the way that the social model of disability has
become a kind of litmus test, by which disability activists assess interventions. If
an initiative or organisation appears to contradict the social model, it must be
rejected as inappropriate, misguided or even oppressive. The simplest form of this
'disability correctness' arises from basic terminology: the social model mandates
the term 'disabled people', because people with impairment are disabled by society,
not by their bodies. The phrase 'people with disabilities' becomes unacceptable
because it implies that 'disabilities' are individual deficits. Those who refer to
'people with disabilities' are thus adopting the 'medical model' and must be re-
educated or repudiated.
     For example, in the late 1990s the UK Government promoted an awareness
campaign intended to challenge discrimination and promote inclusion. A series of

posters of high-achieving disabled people each included the strap line 'See the person not the disability'. The UK disability movement rejected the publicity campaign, largely because it used the term 'disability' to refer to physical impairment (for example Findlay, 1999: 7). There may have been relevant and appropriate criticisms to be made of the 'See the person' campaign. After all, discrimination against disabled people is more than a matter of negative attitudes, and better marketing of disabled people does not seem an adequate response to deep-seated poverty and social exclusion. Yet the disability movement was in danger of giving the impression that the main problem with the Government's approach was that they adopted 'incorrect' terminology.

Many who use the phrase 'people with disabilities' do so because they are striving to be respectful and supportive of disability rights and social inclusion. Rather than defining someone in terms of their impairments, they choose 'people first' terminology to express the common humanity which disabled people share. In other words, while terminology is important, it is not as important as underlying values. Quibbling over 'disabled people' versus 'people with disabilities' is a diversion from making common cause to promote the inclusion and rights of disabled people.

## The unchanging social model

There are several reasons why the social model has now become an obstacle to the further development of the disability movement and disability studies. These reasons are not external to the social model, but intrinsic to its success: the strengths of the social model are also its weaknesses. First, the social model began as the definitions which underpinned a set of practical political positions, from where it became simplified into a series of memorable slogans such as 'disabled by society, not by our bodies'. Developed by ordinary activists, whom Oliver (1990) celebrates as 'organic intellectuals', it was intended to be a political intervention, not a social theory. Politics requires simple and emotionally powerful phrases. The social model was ideally suited to this purpose: it could be explained very quickly, and its implications were obvious and life-transforming.

Second, the social model was developed and promoted in the context of identity politics. For disabled people, the social model was important not just because it highlighted what needed to be changed – the barriers and prejudices and discriminations which they faced daily in their lives – but also because it provided the basis for a stronger sense of identity. Rather than feeling ashamed of impairment, activists could deny that impairment was relevant to their situation. In other words, activists had a strong psychological and emotional attachment to the social model analysis, which became incorporated into their sense of self.

Third, the social model was first devised in the 1970s. It was developed in academic form in the publications of Vic Finkelstein (1980) and Michael Oliver (1990). It was promoted through the work of Colin Barnes (1991) and successive waves of disability studies scholars. Yet at no point in the past thirty years has the social model been developed or revised or rethought. Over and again, the dominant voices of disability studies and the disability movement have reiterated that the fundamental principles of the social model are correct and indispensable (Finkelstein, 2001; Oliver, 2004). Other social movement ideologies such as feminism have developed over time, have contained multiple different inter-pretations and emphases, have responded to criticism and have changed to respond to the changing circumstances, while retaining underlying values. Alone amongst radical movements, the UK disability rights tradition has, like a fundamentalist religion, retained its allegiance to a narrow reading of its founding assumptions.

The goals of the disability movement have always been to promote disability equality and the inclusion of disabled people in society. There is no need for these goals to change. However, the social model is only a means to this end and, as such, it should be revised or replaced if it becomes outdated. There are three central reasons why I now believe that this is the case.

## 1. The impairment/disability distinction

The distinction between impairment and disability lies at the heart of the social model. It is this distinction which separates British disability rights and disability studies from the wider family of social-contextual approaches to disability. Impairment is defined in individual and biological terms. Disability is defined as a social creation. Disability is what makes impairment a problem. For social modellists, social barriers and social oppression constitute disability, and this is the area where research, analysis, campaigning and change must occur.

At first glance, many impairment/disability distinctions appear straightforward. If architects include steps in a building, it clearly disadvantages wheelchair users. Sensory impairments can be remedied by social arrangements such as sign language interpreters, or information in alternative formats. Yet looking closer, the distinction between biological/individual impairment, and social/structural disability is conceptually and empirically very difficult to sustain. Impairments, even sensory impairments, can cause discomfort (Corker and French, 1999: 6). Pain itself is generated through the interplay of physiological, psychological and socio-cultural factors and thus the individual experience can never be separated from the social context (Wall, 1999).

There can be no impairment without society, nor disability without impairment. First, it is necessary to have an impairment to experience disabling barriers. Impairments may not be a sufficient cause of the difficulties which disabled people face, but they are a necessary one. If there is no link between impairment and disability, then disability becomes a much broader, vaguer term which describes any form of socially imposed restriction.

Second, impairments are often caused by social arrangements (Abberley, 1987). For example, a considerable proportion of the global burden of impairment is generated by poverty, malnutrition, war and other collectively or individually imposed social processes. Paul Abberley used this argument to try and deal with the problem of impairment by suggesting that impairment itself could be conceptualised as socially created. Yet because not all impairment is caused by social arrangements, the argument works not to bolster but to undermine the social model. Moreover, impairments are often exacerbated by social arrangements. Environmental and social barriers make impairments worse, both through action and omission. In the first case, having to negotiate physical obstacles, or use badly designed seats or toilets or transport puts people at risk, and may cause pain or injury. In the second case, individuals might experience pain or other symptoms which could be alleviated by drugs or therapies, which are unavailable due to particular prescribing regulations, or to lack of income, or rationing. In each of these cases, are the problems to be defined as socially imposed restriction of activity, or as impairment effects? If social provision was improved, the restriction might disappear, or at least be minimised. But if it wasn't for the impairment, there wouldn't be any restriction in the first place. The problem arises out of the combination of impairment effects and social restrictions.

Third, what counts as impairment is a social judgement. The number of impaired people depends on the definition of what counts as an impairment. The meaning of impairment is a cultural issue, related to values and attitudes of the wider society. The visibility and salience of impairment depend on the expectations and arrangements in a particular society: for example, dyslexia may not become a problem until society demands literacy of its citizens.

What these examples show is that impairment is always already social, while disability is almost always intertwined with impairment effects. Impairment is only ever experienced in a social context. When is a restriction of activity not a social restriction of activity? If disability is defined as social, while impairment is defined as biological, there is a risk of leaving impairment as an essentialist category. Impairment is not a pre-social or pre-cultural biological substrate (Thomas, 1999: 124), as Tremain (2002) has argued in a paper which critiques the untenable ontologies of the impairment–disability and sex–gender distinctions. The words we use and the discourses we deploy to represent impairment are socially and culturally determined. There is no pure or natural body, existing outside of discourse. Impairment is only ever viewed through the lens of disabling social relations. As a crude example, one could cite the labels used to describe a particular impairment: idiocy, mongolism, Down syndrome, trisomy-21 are words which have been used to describe the same impairment situation, yet their connotations differ, as does a generic term such as person with learning difficulties, which might be preferred by many people with that condition

Here, the comparison with feminism is instructive. The early 1970s distinction between sex and gender has been widely criticised by feminist theorists for creating a dangerous dualism of social gender and biological sex. Scholars such as Judith Butler (1990) who have abandoned the sex/gender distinction do not do so in order to return to the traditional idea that woman's being is biological. Instead, it is observed that sex itself is already social. John Hood-Williams concludes his discussion of the problems of dualism by saying:

The sex/gender distinction dramatically advanced understanding in an under-theorised area and, for over twenty years, it has provided a problematic which enabled a rich stream of studies to be undertaken, but it is now time to think beyond its confines.

(Hood-Williams, 1996: 14)

The same, surely, applies to impairment.

In practical terms, the inextricable interconnection of impairment and disability is demonstrated by the difficulty in understanding, in particular examples, where the distinction between the two aspects of disabled people's experience lies. While theoretically or politically it may appear simple to distinguish impairment from disability, qualitative research has found it very difficult to operationalise the social model because it is hard to separate impairment from disability in the everyday lives of disabled people.

For instance, Carol Thomas and Donna Reeve have been pioneers in exploring 'socially engendered undermining of psycho-emotional well being'. For them, this is about extending the social model to show how it is inter-personal encounters and social relations which cause problems, not just physical or economic barriers. This is a helpful development. But, of course, illness and impairment also under-mine psycho-emotional well-being. Having a spinal chord injury or being diagnosed with a degenerative condition can cause depression, anxiety and problems with self-esteem. Thus a person with an impairment may at the same time experience socially engendered psycho-emotional problems, and impairment engendered psycho-emotional problems. In practice, how easy would it be to distinguish between those two causes of mental distress?

For example, consider a person with multiple sclerosis. She might be experiencing psycho-emotional effects for a number of reasons:

1 She may be in pain or suffering other physical symptoms and limitations.
2 She may experience depression as one of the symptoms of the neurological condition itself.
3 She may be experiencing negative reactions from her family, friends and employers, which cause her anger and distress.
4 She may be distressed at the prospect of a disease which will limit her life. This distress may be made worse by the negative cultural representations of MS.
5 She may be experiencing social barriers which make her daily life more of a struggle.
6 She may have other reasons for distress which are unconnected with either the impairment, or the social reaction to it: for example, her cat may have died.

As this individual presents her feelings, how easy it to distinguish the effects of impairment from the effects of disablement (whether defined as barriers or oppression)? What sense would it make to distinguish these different factors in the complexity of an individual psyche? How does 'distress at the prospect of a limiting disease' shade into 'distress at the prospect of a limiting disease which is represented culturally as a fate worse than death'? Could the contribution of the different factors be separated and quantified? It seems likely that the different factors would be inextricably linked, compounding each other in a complex dialectic.

One research project which encountered the difficulty of sustaining the impairment/disability distinction was the doctoral project of Mark Sherry, based on qualitative interviews with people who experienced acquired brain injury (2002). Following a social model approach, Sherry attempted to distinguish between the effects of the injury and the role of barriers or oppression. Yet he was left with a residuum of experiences which could not be classified as either 'impairment' or 'disability' and which he discussed in a chapter called, after Lyotard, 'Different perspectives'. Sherry concluded that impairment and disability experiences and identities were best conceptualised as a fluid continuum, not polar dichotomy.

Another was the study of Lock *et al.* (2005) which took a social model approach to exploring the experience of stroke survivors, finding, 'Predictably, the social model focus on social barriers and social oppression proved to some extent incompatible with the exploration of stroke survivors' experiences' (Lock *et al.* 2005: 34). Their initial focus group data found that respondents experienced impairment effects. 'Difficulties with memory, processing information, speech and language, vision, walking, using the dominant hand and the effects of fatigue were all reported as barriers to employment' (Lock *et al.*, 2005: 43). But of course, they also experienced various disabling barriers:

> Stroke survivors and partners in the focus groups saw their impairments as barriers to work. However, impairments were generally seen as just one element within a complex constellation of actors that act and interact to influence work reintegration.
>
> (Lock *et al.*, 2005: 43)

Another example is offered by Helen Lester and Jonathan Tritter's research with people with serious mental illness: while the authors endorse a social model perspective, their data shows that respondents found it impossible to ignore their impairment and the impact of what 'embodied irrationality'. However, social situations and professional attitudes exacerbated symptoms – what the authors called 'the elision of embodied irrationality and disability' (Lester and Tritter, 2005: 662).

My interpretation of these research studies is that they show the interpenetration of impairment and disability, rather than simply endorsing the social model perspective. In fact, I would argue that any qualitative research with disabled people will inevitably reveal the difficulty of distinguishing impairment and disability (Watson, 2002, 2003).

In responding to criticisms of the social model, Mike Oliver has sought to deal with the problem of impairment by arguing that a social model of impairment is needed alongside the social model of disability (1996: 42). While his recognition of the importance of impairment, and the limitations of the social model, is welcome, it would be neither straightforward nor desirable to make such a distinction, because impairment and disability are not dichotomous. It is difficult to determine where impairment ends and disability starts, but such vagueness need not be debilitating. As I will argue in the next chapter, disability is a complex interaction of biological, psychological, cultural and socio-political factors which cannot be extricated except with imprecision.

## The importance of impairment

> It is not individual limitations, of whatever kind, which are the cause of the problem, but society's failure to provide appropriate services and adequately ensure the needs of disabled people are fully taken into account in its social organisation.
>
> (Oliver, 1996: 32)

The social model defines disability in terms of oppression and barriers, and breaks the link between disability and impairment. This has led to the common criticism that social model approaches have neglected the role of impairment. For example, in her book *Pride Against Prejudice* (1991) Jenny Morris discussed features of disability which had been neglected by the dominant, UPIAS-inspired ideology of the British disability movement: culture, gender, personal identity. Most importantly, she acknowledged that impairment itself created pain and difficulties which were not solely attributable to disabling factors in society:

> While environmental barriers and social attitudes are a crucial part of our experience of disability – and do indeed disable us – to suggest that this is all there is to it is to deny the personal experiences of physical and intellectual restrictions, of illness, of the fear of dying.
>
> (Morris, 1991: 10)

Throughout her book Morris uses disability interchangeably to stand for both social barriers and individual restriction. Following this lead, in 1992 Liz Crow published a paper in *Coalition*, the journal of the Greater Manchester Coalition of Disabled People (subsequently published as Crow, 1996) in which she criticised the social model for failing to encompass the personal experience of pain and limitation which is often a part of impairment. While she expressed commitment to the social model itself, she called for it to be developed in order to find a place for the experience of impairment. She suggested, '[i]nstead of tackling the contradictions and complexities of our experiences head on, we have chosen in our campaigns to present impairment as irrelevant, neutral and, sometimes, positive, but never, ever as the quandary it really is' (Crow, 1996: 208).

Crow did not suggest that impairment was an explanation for disadvantage, but instead that it was an important aspect of disabled people's lives:

As individuals, most of us simply cannot pretend with any conviction that our impairments are irrelevant because they influence every aspect of our lives. We must find a way to integrate them into our whole experience and identity for the sake of our physical and emotional well-being, and, subsequently, for our capacity to work against Disability.

(Crow, 1992: 7)

In the 1993 Open University course book, *Disabling Barriers, Enabling Environments*, Sally French also wrote an important and careful article about the persistence of impairment problems, saying, 'I believe that some of the most profound problems experienced by people with certain impairments are difficult, if not impossible, to solve by social manipulation,' (French, 1993: 17). As a person with visual impairment, she gave the example of being unable to recognise people, and failure to read non-verbal cues in interaction, explaining how these aspects of being a visually impaired person caused problems interacting with neighbours and with her students. According to French, no amount of barrier removal or social change could entirely remedy or remove the problem of visual impairment. French also explored the reasons for resistance to these alternative perspectives:

It is no doubt the case that activists who have worked tirelessly within the disability movement for many years have found it necessary to present disability in a straightforward, uncomplicated manner in order to convince a very sceptical world that disability can be reduced or eliminated by changing society, rather than by attempting to change disabled people themselves.

(French, 1993: 24)

Most recently, Carol Thomas (1999), from within the materialist social model tradition, has developed an approach to disability which makes space for the exploration of personal experience, of the psycho-emotional dimensions of disability, and for the impact of what she calls 'impairment effects'. She uses the latter concept 'to acknowledge that impairments do have direct and restricting impacts on people's social lives' (Thomas, 2004b: 42).

All of these writers have argued from within a social model perspective, calling for reform or development of the model, rather than its abandonment. Nevertheless, many of these critical voices have encountered strong opposition from within the British disability movement and disability studies. Indeed, there has been an implicit tendency to deny the reality of impairment: for example, Dan Goodley seeks to cast doubt on the existence of learning difficulties; 'social structures, practices and relationships continue to naturalise the subjectivities of people with "learning difficulties", conceptualising them in terms of some a priori notion of "mentally impaired"' (Goodley, 2001: 211).

Advocates frequently use scare-quotes and phrases such as 'labelled with learning difficulties'. The BCODP briefing document on the social model refers to 'barriers encountered by people who are viewed by others as having some form of impairment' (British Council of Disabled People, n.d.). Michael Oliver talks of 'people who are viewed by others as having some form of impairment ' (Oliver, 2004). Mental health campaigners use the terminology 'survivors of the mental health system':

> The construct of 'mental illness' is part of a modernist project which devalues the diversity of human experience and perceptions and is preoccupied with analysis, eradication, physicality and mechanical and chemical constraint, rather than understanding, empathy, support and an holistic approach to body and self.
>
> (Beresford and Wallcraft, 1997: 71)

While attention to labelling and discourse is important, there is a danger of ignoring the problematic reality of biological limitation. Linguistic distancing serves as a subtle form of denial.

There are a number of reasons why it might be important for disability studies to engage with impairment:

1   Disability studies should pay attention to the views and perspectives of disabled people, rather than accepting medical claims about the nature and meaning of impairment. Many respondents say that impairment is a central and structuring part of their experience.
2   Disability studies should be concerned with medical responses to impairment. Is treatment effective? Are there side effects? Is research funded effectively? Does the National Health Service prioritise disabled people's impairment needs?
3   Disability studies should be concerned with the prevention of impairment. If there is an interest in the quality of life of disabled people, then this includes minimising the impact of impairment and impairment complications.
4   Disabling barriers both cause and exacerbate impairment. For example, poverty and social exclusion make impairment worse and create additional impairments, particularly risk of mental illness.

Rachel Hurst (2000) makes a familiar comparison of disability to gender, claiming that just as it would be inappropriate to analyse details of women's biology in political debates, so there is no need to analyse individual characteristics of disabled people – 'to concentrate on the personal characteristics of the disabled individual and the functional limitations arising from impairment is itself, disablism' (Hurst, 2000: 1084). It is common to hear such analogies being made between the experiences of disabled people and those of women, minority ethnic communities and lesbians and gays (for example, Gordon and Rosenblum, 2001). For example, Carol Thomas sees the concept 'disablism' as on a par with concepts such as sexism, racism and homophobia. The term 'disablism' has also been deployed by the disability charity, Scope. Perhaps alarmed at being the target of the Direct

Action Network and other disabled rights campaigners, Scope has recently adopted a more radical position, and its campaign 'Time to get equal' is evidence of this. Scope defines 'disablism' as 'discriminatory, oppressive or abusive behaviour arising from the belief that disabled people are inferior to others'. There is an implicit borrowing here from the celebrated definition of institutionalised racism in the Macpherson Report after the death of the black teenager Stephen Lawrence, which included the phrase, 'processes, attitudes and behaviour which amount to discrimination through unwitting prejudice, ignorance, thoughtlessness and racist stereotyping'.

But is the analogy between different movements and oppressions meaningful?

As social movements, women's liberation, gay rights, disability rights and anti-racism are similar in many ways. Each involves identity politics, each challenges the biologisation of difference, each has involved an alliance of academia and activism. There are parallels between the theorisation of disability, and the theorisation of race, gender and sexuality, as the many citations of other oppressions within disability studies literature demonstrate. Yet the oppression which disabled people face is different from, and in many ways more complex than, sexism, racism and homophobia. Women and men may be physiologically and psychologically different, but it is no longer possible to argue that women are made less capable by their biology. 'Gender, like caste, is a matter of social ascription which bears no necessary relation to the individual's own attributes and inherent abilities' (Oakley, 1972: 204).

Similarly, only racists would see the biological differences between ethnic communities as the explanation for their social differences. Nor is it clear why being lesbian or gay would put any individual at a disadvantage, in the absence of prejudice and discrimination. But even in the absence of social barriers or oppression, it would still be problematic to have an impairment, because many impairments are limiting or difficult, not neutral.

Comparatively few restrictions experienced by people with impairment are 'wholly social in origin'. If someone discriminated against disabled people purely because they had an impairment, and imposed exclusions which were solely on this basis and nothing to do with their abilities, then this would be a wholly social restriction. Examples clearly exist of this form of discrimination: nightclubs which exclude disabled people because they cater only to attractive young people; the notorious 'ugly laws' in early twentieth century Chicago and elsewhere which prohibited disfigured people from public spaces. Here, disability discrimination parallels racism, sexism and other social exclusions exactly. But in most cases, disabled people are experiencing both the intrinsic limitation of impairment, and the externally imposed social discrimination.

When disabled people are equated with other historically oppressed groups in a simplistic way, it leads to conclusions which are unwarranted. For example, in her introduction to an important North American collection about disability research, Marcia Rioux argues that once disability is seen as a citizenship issue, traditional research has to change:

> The underlying assumption of the lack of status of persons with disabilities has promoted, or at minimum left unquestioned, the funding and undertaking of research that would be ethically and legally unacceptable if it involved other groups. Studying the genetic make-up of people from non-white racial groups is sceptically viewed. Research into genetic engineering that could be used to prevent female children is sceptically viewed [. . .] Disability ought not to provide a rationale for research that is unacceptable for other groups in society.
>
> (Rioux, 1994: 6)

The implication of the comparison is that genetics is as irrelevant to disabled people as it is to women and non-white ethnic minorities. But this is surely wrong. Unlike the comparator groups, disabled people often experience major disadvantages as a result of their genetic endowment, whereas members of other historically oppressed communities experience either minimal or non-existent biological disadvantages. For a few disabled people, their genetic condition is the most salient aspect of their entire existence.

To take another example, if women or black people have higher rates of unemployment than men or white people, then the explanations might include direct barriers – discrimination by employers – and indirect barriers caused by women and black people lacking appropriate qualifications, training or confidence. However, labour market statistics (Smith and Twomey, 2002) which show that 48 per cent of disabled people of working age are in work compared to 81 per cent of non-disabled people are harder to interpret. Is this disadvantage caused solely by external barriers, or additionally by the particular problems associated with impairment? The 20 per cent of disabled people whose impairments do not limit the kind or amount of work they can do, do not seem to face discrimination. In fact, they are substantially less likely to be unemployed than non-disabled people. The people who are least likely to be working are those with mental illness, of whom only 18 per cent are in work, and those with learning difficulties, of whom only 21 per cent are in work. Some of this can be explained by discrimination, or by the failure of employers to adapt working arrangements to include people with mental illness or learning difficulties. But some of it is because many people with learning difficulties are very limited in the work they can do, and many people with mental health problems find it difficult to cope with regular, stressful work.

The implications of these examples is that impairment often has explanatory relevance in ways that the colour of someone's skin, or their sex, or their sexual orientation usually does not. If social model approaches fail to allow for the role of impairment, they will fail to understand the complexities of disabled people's social situation. Moreover, disability rights academics and activists risk creating stories about disability which many disabled people will not recognise as describing their own experience. As disabled feminists have argued, impairment is an important part of the disability experience. Impairment affects individuals in different ways. Some people are comparatively unaffected by impairment, or else the main consequences of impairment arise from other people's attitudes. For others, impairment limits the experiences and opportunities they can experience. In some cases, impairment causes progressive degeneration and premature death. These features of impairment cause distress to many disabled people, and any adequate account of disability has to give space to the difficulties which many impairments cause. As Simon Williams has argued, 'endorsement of disability solely as social oppression is really only an option, and an erroneous one at that, for those spared the ravages of chronic illness' (Williams, 1999: 812).

Of course, impairment may also lead to opportunities: for example, to experience the world in a different way, or to develop one sense or aptitude because others are unavailable. Moreover everyone, even the supposedly able-bodied, experiences limitations: it's not just the wheelchair user who is unlikely to climb Everest. It is not necessary to claim that all impairments are negative, or that impairment is only and always negative. But for many, impairment is not neutral, because it involves intrinsic disadvantage. Disabling barriers make impairment more difficult, but even in the absence of barriers impairment can be problematic.

## Limitations of the barrier-free world

In his 1980 monograph developing the social model approach pioneered by UPIAS, Vic Finkelstein wrote:

> Once social barriers to the reintegration of people with physical impairments are removed, the disability itself is eliminated. The requirements are for changes to society, material changes to the environment, changes in environmental control systems, changes in social roles, and changes in attitudes by people in the community as a whole.
>
> (Finkelstein, 1980: 33)

Finkelstein (1981) created a powerful fable describing a hypothetical village in which all the inhabitants are wheelchair users, to illustrate the change of emphasis in the barrier philosophy. Everything is adapted to the villagers' needs, and consequently they are not disadvantaged. In other words, they are people with impairments, but not disabled people. When able-bodied people visit the village, it is they who face problems adapting to the environment. They feel excluded, and they experience physical and psychological difficulties. The fable is a powerful summary of the philosophical change which UPIAS demanded, in the form of what would be later known as the social model of disability.

This focus on barriers was carried through into the Open University reader edited by John Swain and colleagues and entitled *Disabling Barriers, Enabling Environments*, and into many documents of the disability rights movement. The global goal of disabled people is a barrier-free world in which disabled people are included, not excluded. In practical terms, the barrier removal mission has radically changed the environment in those countries which have most fully adopted the disability rights critique: for example the United States of America, where barrier removal was mandated by the 1973 Rehabilitation Act section 504 and the 1990 Americans with Disabilities Act. At a slower pace, countries such as the United Kingdom have followed suit.

The barrier removal philosophy underpins the notion of Universal Design, defined by Ron Mace and others as:

> The design of products and environments to be usable by all people, to the greatest extent possible, without the need for adaptation or specialized design.
>
> (Centre for Universal Design, 1997)

The principles of Universal Design were developed by architects, designers and engineers. For example, users should not be stigmatised or segregated: the same means of use should be provided for all users; information should be in multiple formats and accessible to all; design should be usable with low physical effort; size and space should be appropriate for users with different body sizes, seated or standing. Rob Imrie (2004) has welcomed the development of Universal Design, while expressing caution about its limitations: for example, social and economic relations play a major role in disabling people, and it is not enough to address buildings and products without addressing money and power.

Despite Finklestein's fable and the development of Universal Design, limited conceptual work has been done on the concept of the barrier-free world. There are so many obvious barriers yet to be removed, that perhaps it has not seemed necessary to think too hard about what the inclusive environment might look like, when the utopia is finally achieved. But thinking about a barrier-free utopia is vital for those seeking to conceptualise disability, because the social model is predicated on the assumption that it is possible to remove the barriers which disable people with impairment (although of course the philosophy of barrier removal is not limited to social model perspectives, being present in most social-contextual accounts of disability).

Ironically, the very success of many developed nations in developing inclusive public spaces may provide new evidence that the barriers model is not a sufficient explanation of disability. First, as the obvious and unnecessary barriers are removed, the more stubborn and complex exclusions are left in greater relief, and the deeper moral and political questions about priorities and cost-effectiveness become starker. Second, if disabled people remain poor and disadvantaged, despite social and environmental change, then it suggests that a civil rights or social model philosophy may not be the full solution to the problem of disability. For example, while the United States of America has strong civil rights legislation, which has mandated the most accessible environment in the world, disabled Americans remain disproportionately poor, and many are forced to live in segregated nursing homes (Russell, 2002).

Perhaps it is unfair to judge the social model approach on the validity of the concept of the barrier-free world. After all, the social model is about more than physical environments. The BCODP states that the barriers disabled people encounter include inaccessible education systems, working environments, inadequate disability benefits, discriminatory health and social support systems, inaccessible transport, houses and public buildings and amenities, and the devaluing of disabled people through negative images in the media.

(British Council of Disabled People, n.d.)

Architectural and communications barrier removal is often easier than the removal of social and economic barriers. Progress on many of these latter issues has been much slower to achieve, which may explain the persisting poverty of disabled people. After all, minority ethnic groups and women have faced few if any architectural barriers, yet still remain disadvantaged and excluded due to institutional discrimination, the glass ceiling and other insidious social and economic disadvantages. Seeking to reclaim a relational interpretation, Carol Thomas highlights the ways in which the early social model literature stresses oppression as the defining feature of disability. For example, following UPIAS' definition of disability as restriction quoted earlier comes the phrase: 'disabled people are therefore an oppressed group in society'. Thomas (2004a) claims that rather than focusing on barriers, social modellists should focus on relations of oppression.

Conceding that physical obstacles are only a part of the barriers and oppression which disabled people face, a focus on environmental barriers is justified for two reasons. First, creating an accessible environment would reduce social exclusion. Second, the physical obstacles approach to understanding how people are disabled has a powerful symbolic role. The conventional view of disabled people focuses on what people with impairments cannot do, physically: for example, not being able to walk or see or hear. The social model has stressed that this deficit approach is wrong, because using a wheelchair or Braille or sign language is not inferior to the majority approaches to mobility or communication, just different. Using a wheelchair only becomes a problem because the world has been badly designed or unfairly built. In other words, ideas about performance, deficit and access are key to the popular understandings of disability which the social model seeks to challenge. Problems with the notion of barrier removal therefore provide objections to the social model concept itself.

## Problems with the barrier-free utopia

### Nature

The claim that people are disabled by society, not by their bodies, has been effective in highlighting the human-created obstacles to participation in society. Yet outside the city the social model seems harder to implement. Wheelchair users are disabled by sandy beaches and rocky mountains. People with visual impairments may be unable to see a sunset, and people with hearing impairments will miss out on the sounds of birds, wind and waves. It is hard to blame the natural environment on social arrangements.

Of course, benign social arrangements can mitigate some of these exclusions (Tregaskis, 2004b). A paved path or wooden walkway can enable people with mobility restrictions to access nature reserves, sites of natural beauty and historic monuments. The use of video cameras and audio description will go some way to opening up inaccessible nature. Yet inevitably people with impairments will always be disadvantaged by their bodies: they will not be able to climb every mountain. Even if it were practically possible, it would defeat the very idea of wilderness to create roads and other access facilities to unspoilt and inaccessible landscapes.

Within urban areas, it is possible to make both private homes and public buildings accessible. Yet if a wheelchair user lives on top of a hill, then they will face major barriers to getting around their local environment. Some cities – for example San Francisco – are innately less accessible than others – for example Cambridge. Equally, wheelchair users in the Nordic countries are regularly disabled by snowfall, whereas their counterparts in southerly latitudes can negotiate the streets throughout the winter months.

## Incompatibility

Implicit in the notion of a barrier-free world is the idea that Universal Design can liberate all. Yet, while in each case a solution to an access barrier can often be found, taken as a totality it may be impossible to create one environment which is accessible for all potential users. The principles of Universal Design are unarguable when taken separately, but may create conflict when aggregated.

For example, wheelchair users demand level access. Yet people with mobility issues who do not use wheelchairs may find that steps are safer and easier for them than ramps. Blind people may find that kerb cuts which liberate wheelchair users make it difficult for them to differentiate pavement from road, and leave them vulnerable to walking into the path of a vehicle. Wheelchair users may have problems with tactile paving which gives locational cues to visually impaired people (Grey-Thompson, 2005). Partially sighted people may request large text on white background: people with dyslexia may prefer black print on yellow paper. Some people will prefer rooms to be dim, others will prefer them to be brightly lit.

Moreover, different people with the same impairment may require different accommodation, because everyone experiences their own impairment differently, and each impairment comes in different forms, and different people have different preferences for solving impairment problems. Surveying 1,000 Americans' views on domestic adaptation, Stark (2001) found

> the solution to environmental problems is highly individual for each person and will result from a plan that includes multiple strategies (including architectural modification, assistive technology, programmatic support, and personal support), and considers the perspective of the individual.

> (Stark, 2001: 47)

Some people with visual impairment prefer to access information in large print, others use Braille, and others prefer to access information on audio tape or on computer disc. In other words, fully accessible information would come in a range of different formats, suitable for different users (Imrie, 2004: 282; French, 1993). Barrier removal might mean making every library book available in every format. When consideration is given to expense, person time and storage space, this solution seems inefficient and impractical. In practice, an easier solution would be to use computer technology: new books could be provided to the library as computer files, and a machine could output the information via a voice synthesiser, or a brailler, or a computer screen, depending on the individual preference of the visually impaired or indeed dyslexic user. Such an approach would make some of the information contained in the library accessible on demand, and possibly give the disabled user equal access to the non-disabled user. Disabled users would achieve the same ends as non-disabled users, but via separate and specific and possibly segregated means. This may contain the spirit of a barrier-free environment, but perhaps not the universal utopia which some rhetoric imagines. Measures of this kind begin to sound like a response to special needs, not an inclusive and non-discriminatory universal provision.

### Practicality

The library example begins to highlight problems of practicality which may mean that it is impossible to remove every obstacle. For example, it may be considered a poor use of resources to provide books in multiple formats, if this reduces the budget for buying new books. It may be more practical to undertake to make any book available if specifically requested within a reasonable timeframe. This again moves closer to special and separate provision than the concept of a barrier-free world, but may seem to many authorities to be a reasonable and practical compromise.

Another area where principles may be less useful than pragmatism concerns buildings and facilities which were constructed in an era where the participation of disabled people was never considered. For example, the New York subway and the London underground are largely inaccessible to wheelchair users, unlike the more modern transit systems in Washington and Newcastle, each of which was built with elevators and ramps to accommodate the full range of users. Clearly, principles of Universal Design demand that new buildings are barrier-free. But debate rages as to whether authorities are obliged to make accessible existing facilities, where retro-fitting would impose huge costs and simpler measures to facilitate the independent transport of disabled people could be found. For example, Transport for London runs almost 100 per cent accessible buses. Consequently, disabled people can use public transport, but cannot make a choice between underground and bus transport. They can achieve the same ends as non-disabled people but do not have the same freedom of means. The transport system is not fully accessible, but arguably it is accessible enough to ensure dignified, non-segregated transit.

Fully accessible and barrier-free facilities are an important goal, but there are huge difficulties to achieving them. For example, finding accessible facilities for the annual UK disability studies conferences has proved extremely difficult. Financial constraints mean that a university campus is the only realistic possibility. It is far from straightforward to find a campus which can accommodate up to 200 disabled people. In practice, access is often a compromise, and depends on goodwill and flexibility.

### Barrier removal means rebuilding society

The implications of creating a fully accessible society are very far reaching. For example, it might mean not just accessible transport, information and public buildings, but also accessible private homes. At the moment, it is a struggle for many disabled people to find accessible accommodation for themselves. This is a major civil rights issue, and a indictment of the failure of many societies to remove barriers or to build effective provision. Land is scarce, and hence at a premium, in the United Kingdom. Single storey dwellings are rare, and disproportionately expensive. Many bungalows are designed with older people in mind, and as a consequence do not have the number of bedrooms or size of rooms to suit either a young family, or someone manoeuvring a wheelchair. Even those with access to finance find it difficult to locate a suitable property for purchase. It is not far-fetched to think that something could be done about this. Developers could be encouraged to build a higher number of single storey or accessible homes within new build developments. It could be made a condition of receiving planning permission, or subsidies could be made available to reduce the cost of such dwellings. Housing associations are another way of making low cost accessible houses available. In this way, it could be made much easier for disabled people to find appropriate accommodation (Madigan and Milner, 1999).

But in an ideal barrier-free world, a disabled person would not just be able to rely on her own home being fully accessible, but would also be able to visit her friends. The minimum requirement would be able to enter the ground floor in order to socialise, and have access to a toilet. Brief consideration of the UK shows how difficult it would be to achieve this. Most of the housing stock in the UK is not new build, and the vast majority presents barriers to people who use wheelchairs. A major transformation seems unlikely, but with political will, new build homes could be forced to conform to 'Lifetime Housing' standards. However, for the foreseeable future, a wheelchair user will find that most of her friends and relatives live in homes which she is unable to access.

Thinking about other disabled people, there are similar problems. Some people experience impairments which cause pain and fatigue. Barrier-free environments and mobility aids may make it easier for them to negotiate the world. But they may still be immensely limited, and perhaps unable to participate directly in social or economic activities. Even in a barrier-free world, they may remain confined largely to their own homes, or unable to work for more than a few hours a day and hence excluded from the world of work, even if they have the intellectual abilities to contribute.

Imagining how a barrier-free world might be achieved for people with learning difficulties. Short of a global catastrophe which returned western society to medieval levels of economic and social organisation, it would be impossible to recreate a world in which literacy and numeracy were not important attributes for economic independence and advancement. Clearly, many people with learning difficulties have basic literacy and numeracy skills, and there are good examples of people living independently and engaging in paid work. Creating better sheltered and supported employment possibilities to enable people with learning difficulties to benefit from the income, self-esteem and social integration which jobs provide should be a priority for any disability policy (Gosling and Cotterill, 2000). Yet a significant proportion of people with learning difficulties have little prospect of performing even basic work tasks (Vehmas, 2006).

Thinking more specifically still, Judy Singer (1999) asks what barrier removal might mean for people with social impairments such as autism? If someone's impairment makes interaction with others difficult, it is difficult to see how the mainstream world could be adapted to accommodate him alongside other people. People could be educated to become more accepting and supportive of people with autism: this would remove one source of distress and cruelty. But someone with autism may find even the most well-meaning and respectful crowd of people still a disturbing and confusing invasion. With imagination, perhaps facilities could have special sessions reserved for people with social impairments, where people could shop or swim or learn without feeling crowded or disturbed by the presence of others. But again, this begins to sound less like barrier-free provision, and more like the specialised and perhaps even segregated provision of solutions for special needs. Ultimately, some people with autism may prefer self-exclusion to inclusion.

Advocating enabling spatial organisation, Peter Freund (2001) asks how much difference can be accommodated. While limitations of the body will always remain restricting, he argues that there are many unexplored avenues for accomodating different 'mind-bodies'. This reconstruction of space would benefit many bodies, not just those with impairments. I find Freund's analysis helpful, and it is not my intention to oppose barrier removal in practice. But on a theoretical level, the barrier-removal solution to disability does not fully succeed, and this failure undermines the tenets of the social model. Neil Levy (2002: 139) argues that for a social causation model of disability to work, two conditions must apply: first, it must be possible to alter social arrangements so as to remove disadvantage and second, there must be no compelling reason why social arrangements could not be altered. Resource constraints are sometimes a compelling reason preventing the removal of barriers. The specifics of impairment also create disadvantage which no inclusive social arrangements can mitigate. In these situations provision of alternative ways of accessing facilities or services can often be both appropriate and acceptable.

The disability rights movement has always worked for inclusive provision and a barrier-free world. But barrier removal is not an ends in itself. It is a means to an end. The aim of barrier removal is to facilitate the participation and improve the quality of life of people with impairment. In many cases, barrier removal and inclusive provision are the most appropriate and cost-effective ways of achieving that end, with the added advantage of minimising segregation of disabled from non-disabled people. But sometimes separate or alternative provision for disabled people may be a more appropriate way of enabling them to achieve their ends and goals. For example, for people with autism that might be about providing spaces and opportunities for them to work, shop, learn or socialise where there are fewer people, fewer disturbing sounds or images, less disruption and more routine. For people with learning difficulties, that might be about supported living or working situations, or learning opportunities, or alternatives to employment which give a sense of value, purpose and fulfilment to their lives.

## Conclusion

The social model of disability makes a distinction between impairment and disability; claims that disability can be removed by social change; and downplays the role of impairment in the lives of disabled people. In this chapter, I have argued against each of these points. My claim is that, even in the most accessible world, there will always be residual disadvantage attached to many impairments. If people have fatigue, there is a limited amount that can be done to help: motorised scooters and other aids may help increase range and scope of activities, but ultimately the individual will be disadvantaged, when compared to others. Sally French, in her discussion of visual impairment, argues that providing adapted equipment and information to people with visual impairment does not remove disabling barriers, and may even make them worse by removing human contact (French, 1993: 19).

The concepts of a barrier-free world and of Universal Design are immensely valuable in highlighting the many ways in which unnecessary barriers and thoughtless planning disadvantages many people with impairment, or who have dependents, or who are old or injured. There is undoubtedly a moral and political imperative to do much more to promote inclusion. But there are major practical and intrinsic obstacles to solving the problem of disability solely or perhaps even chiefly through barrier removal. As Michael Bury has argued, 'The reduction of barriers to participation does not amount to abolishing disability as a whole' (Bury, 1997: 137).

Underlying the idea of a barrier-free world is an attempt to show that impairments can be irrelevant, and to equalise disabled and non-disabled people. Those who adopt the social model are relativist, in that they claim that having an impairment is a different but equal form of embodiment to not having an impairment. From a social model perspective, it is not the form of embodiment which is the problem, but the failure of the social world to accommodate to that form of embodiment by removing barriers. Various examples or folktales are deployed to illustrate this insight. For example, Michael Oliver has claimed that 'An aeroplane is a mobility aid for non-flyers in exactly the same way as a wheelchair is a mobility aid for non-walkers' (Oliver, 1996: 108). This sort of statement is amusing, provocative, and forces people to attend to the ways in which we take certain things for granted. But it cannot be taken seriously. Not being able to fly is not the equivalent of not being able to walk. While both aeroplanes and wheelchairs enable individuals to overcome the natural restrictions of their bodies, walking is part of normal species functioning for human beings, whereas flying is not. There is no symmetry or equality between the situation of the non-flyer and the non-walker. A wheelchair is not just one travel option for a paralysed person: it is an essential facilitator.

A second example is the frequent reference to Nora Groce's historical study of Martha's Vineyard. In this isolated community in America, deafness was common. It is argued that because Deaf people could communicate with all their neighbours, they did not experience disabling barriers, and hearing impairment was not a problem. Like Oliver's flyers and wheelers, this is a suggestive and valuable lesson for those who refuse to accept that disability can be normalised. But it is not evidence that a barrier-free environment eliminates disability and equalises non-disabled and disabled people. Deaf Vineyarders may have flourished in their isolated community, but unless all their hearing companions were to forgo speech, they would still miss out on some social interaction. Hearing people would have had the advantage of two forms of communication, speech and sign language, whereas Deaf people would have been limited to one form of communication, however effective. They would not have had the same choices as their hearing companions to leave the community and trade or travel off-island. They would have been disadvantaged in experiencing and negotiating the natural world because of the lack of one of their major senses.

Finkelstein's utopian village provides a third example, and is similarly an illusory solution to the disability problem. Moreover, by equating able-bodied with disabled people, it glosses a real disadvantage. No village for wheelchair users would be inaccessible to non-disabled people, for the simple reason that non-disabled people always have the choice to use wheelchairs, just as hearing people have the choice to learn sign language. Again, there is no symmetry. These examples imply something important about the difference between disabled people and non-disabled people. Disabled people have less flexibility and fewer choices than non-disabled people. As Janet Radcliffe Richards has put it, an ability cannot be turned into a disability, just as no change of values turns a disability into an ability. An accessible environment minimises the inconvenience of impairment, but does not equalise disabled people with non-disabled people.

Those who defend the social model, and see no reason for it to be revised or replaced, will remain unpersuaded. In particular, they will claim that my analysis creates a 'straw person'. I have misinterpreted the social model, and given an inaccurate picture of how people in the disability movement really think and operate. Nobody seeks to deny the body or impairment. Nobody is opposed to medical intervention (Oliver, 2004). There are no crude dichotomies.

There are three responses to this defence. First, I have cited examples above – and there are many more – when the public position and campaigns of the disability movement have promoted exactly the sorts of positions and distinctions which I criticise. Academic defenders of the social model are trying to have it both ways. They protest that they are not promoting crude dichotomies with one breath, whereas with the other they do exactly what they are disavowing. While some of the leading exponents of the social model now claim to operate a less rigid approach, they still simultaneously reinforce the 'strong' social model. Second, it may be true that, in private, activists don't consistently think or talk in terms of the social model. For example, many disability rights campaigners concede that behind closed doors they talk about aches and pains and urinary tract infections, even while they deny any relevance of the body while they are out campaigning. Yet this inconsistency is surely wrong: if the public rhetoric says one thing, while everyone behaves privately in a more complex way, then perhaps it is time to re-examine the rhetoric and speak more accurately. For example, Kirsten Stalker *et al.* (1999) found that many voluntary organisations which claimed to support the social model in practice used concepts which were incompatible with it. Rather than condemning their inconsistencies, I would applaud the pragmatism of people working in the field: the problem is the limitations of a model which is hard to operationalise.

Alternatively, defenders of the social model orthodoxy will argue that it is unfair to criticise the inadequacies of the social model, because it is not a fully fledged social theory. For example, Vic Finkelstein has said:

> In my view juvenile criticisms of the social model of disability arise because it is frequently used as if it explains our situation rather than as a tool for gaining insight into the way that society disables us . . . The social model does not explain what disability is. For an explanation we would need a social theory of disability.
>
> (Finkelstein, 2001: 10)

Similarly, Michael Oliver has argued that 'the social model of disability is a practical tool, not a theory, an idea or a concept.' (2004: 30) and that 'models are ways of translating ideas into practice' (2004: 19). Oliver also suggests that 'it seems superfluous to criticise the social model for not being something that it has never claimed to be' (2004: 24).

It is hard to know how to respond to these defences of the social model. The social model certainly provides a definition of disability. According to the Concise Oxford Dictionary, 'definition' means 'stating precise form of thing or meaning of word' whilst the most relevant definition of 'model' is as 'simplified description of system'. The distinctions between the social model as definition, as explanation, as a tool for insight, as a tool for practice, or as a social theory do not seem significant to me. Llewellyn and Hogan (2000) argue that a model is usually a small-scale theory to promote understanding and generate new research hypotheses. But the social model of disability seeks to have a larger application, and it is misleading to see it as a model. Instead, they suggest that it should be seen as a theoretical system:

> A system is a general theory in the grand sense, it seeks to describe what the subject of study is about, as well as commenting on the methods that should be employed to research into it. A system, then, needs to be inclusive in that it seeks to account for a wide range of phenomena, organises the available data and offers an account of this.
>
> (Llewellyn and Hogan, 2000: 164)

Social model advocates freely criticise accounts of disability which are not based on the social model. Yet they resist criticism on the basis that the social model is not a social theory or an explanation or an idea. Again, advocates of the social model are trying to have it both ways. After thirty years of writing about the social model and applying the social model, it is hard to deny that the social model provides a theoretical system or paradigm, however much this label is abjured. Above all, it hardly matters whether the social model is a system, model, paradigm, idea, definition or even tool. What matters is that the social model is wrong.

# Chapter 4

# Disability

## A complex interaction

Earlier, I challenged the assumption that the social model was the only progressive or social-contextual approach to disability, and then demonstrated why I believe that the social model fails as a conceptualisation of disability. If disability studies scholars and activists are to abandon the social model, then an alternative social-contextual approach is needed which can reconcile different aspects of disability, and serve as the basis for a progressive politics. In this chapter, I make an initial contribution to that endeavour.

First, I should state my theoretical allegiance. In my work, I have found a plurality of approaches beneficial in the analysis of disability. For example feminism offers the concept of the personal being political; Foucault highlights the medical gaze, and the genealogical method; post-structuralism deconstructs notions of identity; postmodernism challenges binary dichotomies and opens up space for complexity; Ian Hacking critiques social constructionism and explores how different ways of conceptualising categories change people's possibilities for self-understanding (Hacking, 2000). The work of Nancy Fraser (1995, 2000) and Axel Honneth (1995) has proved powerful in explaining the demands of radical social movements, and the different dimensions of oppression. Rather than tie myself to one view or model, I have tried to take useful elements from different theorists. This selectivity may lead to inconsistency, but avoids the danger of trying to fit the complexities and the nuances of life into an over-rigid structure or system. In order to put my ontological cards onto the theoretical table, I should state now that I find the critical realist perspective to be the most helpful and straightforward way of understanding the social world, because it allows for this complexity.

Critical realism means acceptance of an external reality: rather than resorting to relativism or extreme constructionism, critical realism attends to the independent existence of bodies which sometimes hurt, regardless of what we may think or say about those bodies. Critical realists distinguish between ontology (what exists) and epistemology (our ideas about what exists). They believe that there are objects independent of knowledge: labels describe, rather than constitute, disease. In other words, while different cultures have different views or beliefs or attitudes to disability, impairment has always existed and has its own experiential reality. Within disability research, strong statements from the critical realist perspective have been made by Simon Williams (1999) and Danermark and Gellerstedt (2004). Both seek to avoid arguments over medical model versus social model perspectives by demanding an approach that gives weight to different causal levels in the complex disability experience. For example, Williams concludes:

> Disability . . . is an emergent property, located, temporally speaking, in terms of the interplay between the biological reality of physiological impairment, structural conditioning (i.e. enablements/constraints) and socio-cultural interaction/elaboration.
>
> (Williams, 1999: 810)

whereas Danermark and Gellerstedt suggest:

> This implies that injustices to disabled people can be understood neither as generated by solely cultural mechanisms (cultural reductionism) nor by socio-economic mechanisms (economic reductionism) nor by biological mechanisms (biological reductionism). In sum, only by taking different levels, mechanisms and contexts into account, can disability as a phenomenon be analytically approached.
>
> (Danermark and Gellerstedt, 2004: 350)

The critical realist perspective appears to offer a good basis on which to elaborate a workable understanding of disability, which combines the best aspects of both the traditional and the radical accounts.

## Disability as an interaction

According to those who follow the social model (Oliver, 1990; Barnes, 1998b), traditional accounts of disability have been individual and medical in their focus. The alternative social model of disability is a structural and social approach, emphasising barriers and oppression. While the UK disability movement has endorsed the social model perspective, academic dissenting voices have been raised both within (Morris, 1991; Crow, 1996; French, 1993) and outside (Williams, 1999) the disability studies community. These criticisms have centred on the failure of the social model to recognise the role of impairment, as well as the inability of the social model to encompass the range of different impairment/disability experiences.

The approach to disability which I propose to adopt suggests that disability is always an interaction between individual and structural factors. Rather than getting fixated on defining disability either as a deficit or a structural disadvantage, a holistic understanding is required. The experience of a disabled person results from the relationship between factors intrinsic to the individual, and extrinsic factors arising from the wider context in which she finds herself. Among the intrinsic factors are issues such as: the nature and severity of her impairment, her own attitudes to it, her personal qualities and abilities, and her personality. Among the contextual factors are: the attitudes and reactions of others, the extent to which the environment is enabling or disabling, and wider cultural, social and economic issues relevant to disability in that society.

The difference between my interactional approach and the social model is that while I acknowledge the importance of environments and contexts, including discrimination and prejudice, I do not simply define disability as the external disabling barriers or oppression. I thus avoid what Mårten Söder calls 'contextual essentialism'. The problems associated with disability cannot be entirely eliminated by any imaginable form of social arrangements. The priority for a progressive disability politics is to engage with impairment, not to ignore it.

The difference between my approach and what social modellists would describe as the medical model is that I do not explain disability solely in terms of impairment. My approach is non-reductionist, because I accept that limitations are always experienced as an interplay of impairment with particular contexts and environments. Impairment is a necessary but not sufficient factor in the complex interplay of issues which results in disability. Social modellists would claim that 'medical modellists' assume that 'people are disabled by their bodies', whereas they say instead that 'people are disabled by society, not by their bodies'. I would argue that 'people are disabled by society and by their bodies'.

There are similarities beween my interactional approach and the relational model adopted by Carol Thomas (1999). She developed her amended version of the social model as a result of the qualitative research she carried out with disabled women. This led her to add the concept of 'impairment effects' to the dualistic conception of impairment and disability which Oliver had outlined. This concept allows Thomas to account for individual limitations which arise from impairment, rather than from social oppression. Thomas has also made two other innovations. First, she argued that disability (by which she means social oppression) has psycho-emotional effects. This I agree with, although I would add that impairment also has psycho-emotional effects. Second, she argued that the original UPIAS approach should be understood relationally, and that disability should be defined in terms of oppression rather than barriers. She distinguishes (2004a, 2004b) between what she sees as the original UPIAS social relational understanding and the subsequent social model of disability. Thomas equates the social model with a stress on barriers to activity and believes that it is this which has caused the confusion over impairment.

However, in my opinion Thomas has falsely made a distinction between a social oppression and a social barriers version of the social model. Both aspects co-exist in both the UPIAS formulation and the subsequent development of the social model.

Thomas appears to be trying to refine, develop and tweak the social model to deal with the absences, limitations and confusions to which it leads. While she now suggests that the social model should be set to one side (2004b: 33), she does not want to abandon it. Although for her it is not a 'credible social interpretation of disability', she believes it is of symbolic importance both because it differentiates disability studies from medical sociology, and orients disability studies to the disability movement.

Thomas and I both agree that a relational approach to understanding disability is needed. By relational, I mean that the disability is a relationship between intrinsic factors (impairment, etc.) and extrinsic factors (environments, support systems, oppression, etc.). However, Thomas uses the term 'social relational' to refer to the relationship of 'those socially constructed as problematically different because of a significant bodily and/or cognitive variation from the norm and those who meet the cultural criteria of embodied normality' (Thomas, 2004b: 28).

While recognition of the role of power is important for any theory of disability, Thomas' approach is fatally flawed because it defines disability (and hence disabled people) in terms of oppression – 'Disability is a form of social oppression involving the social imposition of restrictions of activity on people with impairments and the socially engendered undermining of their psycho-emotional wellbeing' (Thomas, 1999: 60).

There are a number of problems with this claim:

1   Thomas reproduces the circularity within the traditional social model. If disability is defined in terms of oppression, then this puts social researchers into a difficult position. When researching disability, they are committed to finding that disabled people are oppressed, by definition. The only question is the extent to which disabled people are oppressed. Anders Gustavsson (2004: 67) quotes Mårten Söder arguing that this circular reasoning is a particular danger of either clinical or contextual essentialism.

2   It seems that Thomas is further committed to separating two categories: the set of people with impairment (who may experience impairment effects) and within that the subset of disabled people (meaning people with impairment who experience oppressive social reactions in addition to their impairment effects). For example, I may not consider myself to be oppressed much of the time: I certainly have an impairment, and sometimes environments, policies or social reactions are oppressive and damaging to my psycho-emotional wellbeing. Often, however, they are not. In other words, in some situations I am a person with impairment, and in other situations I am a disabled person, according to Thomas' definitions. This seems impractical and confusing.

3   Many disabled people, much of the time, actually experience positive responses from non-disabled people. For example, they may receive support from non-disabled relatives, friends, or strangers who assist them in daily activities. Or they may experience positive benefit from statutory or voluntary services. To define disability entirely in terms of oppression risks obscuring the positive dimension of social relations which enable people with impairment.

Note the difference between the impairment/disability distinction, and the sex/gender distinction with which it is often compared. Feminists (for example Oakley

1972) distinguished between biological sex (male/female) and socio-cultural gender (masculine/feminine). They argued that to be a man or woman in a particular historical and cultural context was a social, not a biological, experience. Yet they did not claim that gender equalled oppression, even though they provided evidence that women had historically been oppressed in different ways. Gender was socio-cultural, and often associated with oppression. Compare Thomas' view of disability: impairment is defined, in the social model, as an individual biological attribute (corresponding to sex for the feminists). But the social model does not define disability as the socio-cultural experience of impairment. Instead, disability is defined as oppression – or in Thomas' phrase 'forms of oppressive social reaction visited upon people with impairments' (2004b: 579).

Thomas argues (2004b) that I am committed to a commonplace meaning of disability as 'not being able to do things' and as 'restricted activity'. I deny her interpretation of the position outlined in Shakespeare and Watson (2001a). Then, as now, I define disability as the outcome of the interaction between individual and contextual factors – which includes impairment, personality, individual attitudes, environment, policy, and culture. Rather than reserving the word disability for 'impairment effects' or 'oppression' or 'barriers', I would rather use the term broadly to describe the whole interplay of different factors which make up the experience of people with impairments. Impairment is a necessary but not sufficient element in the disability relationship. It is always the combination of a certain set of physical or mental attributes, in a particular physical environment, within a specified social relationship, played out within a broader cultural and political context, which combines to create the experience of disability for any individual or group of individuals (Sim et al., 1998). I am happy to accept that both social barriers and oppression play a part in generating disability for many disabled people in many contexts. But I cannot accept that disability should be defined as either social barriers or oppression.

I would not claim to have a wholly new and original understanding of disability. The obviousness of my conception is one of its merits, and others have argued very similar things (Williams, 1999; Danermark and Gellerstedt, 2004; Gabel and Peters, 2004). For example, the Nordic relational approach corresponds closely to my understanding of disability: Anders Gustavsson talks about the relative interactionist perspective as an alternative to essentialism, 'a theoretical perspective that rejects assumptions about any primordial analytical level and rather takes a programmatic position in favor of studying disability on several different analytical levels' (Gustavsson, 2004: 62).

A recent paper by van den Ven and a Dutch team (van den Ven et al., 2005) came to a similar conclusion based on qualitative research. They concluded:

Both the individual with a disability and others in society have a shared responsibility with respect to the integration of people with disabilities into society. Each must play their part for integration to occur: it takes two to tango. An individual with a disability should be willing to function in society and adopt an attitude towards others in society in such a way that they can join in with activities and people in society. On the other hand society should take actions to make functioning in society possible for people with disabilities. In other words, society should be inclusive with respect to people with disabilities by passing laws on anti-discrimination, ensuring accessibility of buildings and arranging appropriate care facilities for people with disabilities.

(Van den Ven *et al.*, 2005: 324)

These authors, like myself, balance medical and social aspects. They refer to three issues which influence integration: individual factors, which include personality and skills as well as impairment; societal factors, referring to accessibility, attitudes, etc.; and factors within the system of support, by which they mean social support, professional care and assistive devices. The interrelation of these three sets of factors determine or produce disability. This research team adopt a conception of integration which I also find helpful. They highlight five elements:

1   Functioning in an ordinary way without getting special attention or being singled out as a result of disability.
2   Mixing with others and not being ignored in friendship and networks.
3   Taking part in and contributing to society whether through paid work or volunteering.
4   Trying to realise one's potential – which may need help from others.
5   Being director of one's life.

This approach seems adequate to the complexity and diversity of disabled people and their aspirations, and a helpful basis for future research.

Thomas (2004a) is right to suggest that there are no contradictions between my own understanding and that of Williams or Bury, or indeed of the WHO's International Classification of Functioning, Disability and Health (ICF). The medico-psycho-social model which lies at the heart of the ICF does seem to me a sensible and practical way of understanding the complexity of disability. Some disability rights commentators have rejected the new WHO framework as being no more than a rebadging of the discredited International Classification of Impairments, Disabilities and Handicaps (Pfeiffer, 1998, 2000; Hurst, 2000). Yet the new approach does recognise the role of the environment in causing restriction (Imrie, 2004). It does not use the term 'disability' to refer to either impairment, functional limitation, or indeed environmental barriers, but uses it to describe the entire process:

the locus of the problem and the focus of intervention are situated not solely within the individuals, but also within their physical, social and attitudinal environments. The label of disability becomes a description of the outcome of the interaction of the individual and the environnment and not merely a label applied to a person.

(Bornman, 2004: 186)

Following Zola (1989), the ICF framers recognise that the entire population is at risk of impairment and its consequences (Bickenbach *et al.*, 1999). While Rob Imrie (2004) is correct to note that the ICF is theoretically underdeveloped, for all these reasons I believe that it offers a way forward for defining and researching disability, and should be endorsed by disability studies.

An interactional model is able to account for the range and diversity of disability experiences. For example, there can be variation depending on the nature and extent of the impairment. Simo Vehmas (2006) has written about Steve, a man with profound intellectual impairments. Steve cannot communicate or live independently, let alone work. However, he can respond to certain stimuli and can express pleasure and pain. Vehmas argues that Steve will not be helped by initiatives such as independent living, civil rights or barrier removal: they will not make a difference to his life, because his impairment is so limiting. Any social theory of disability has to avoid the error of conflating the variety of disabled people's experience. Impairment is scalar and multi-dimensional, and differences in impairment contribute to the level of social disadvantage which individuals face.

Failure to appreciate the impairment continuum contributes to some of the sterile arguments about the nature of disability. It appears to me that some of those who see disability as a tragedy which should be prevented at all costs are seeing only the most severe end of the continuum. And some of those who deny that impairment can be problematic, and see disability as just another difference, are seeing only the milder end of the continuum. In other words, the two camps are talking at cross purposes: because they think of different cases when they discuss disability, they are unable to come to agreement about how disability should be understood or defined.

A related phenomenon is the distinction which disability studies theorists have attempted to draw between chronic illness and impairment. This appears to be an attempt to reject the critique of medical sociologists such as Michael Bury, Gareth Williams and Michael Kelly (Barnes and Mercer, 1996). It also shores up the social model by emphasising disabled people who have static conditions which do not degenerate or need medical care. But in practice it is hard to say that people with multiple sclerosis, HIV/AIDS or cystic fibrosis are not disabled people, and it has been important to include such conditions in disability discrimination legislation. For some individuals impairment is a major limiting factor, which renders any social manipulation or barrier removal almost irrelevant. For others, impairment itself causes little restriction: it is the reaction of others which causes problems of exclusion and disadvantage. The interactional model can allow for this variation.

One of the reasons why disability rights activists and disability studies have been unwilling to look too closely at the issue of impairment differences is perhaps the fear of reinforcing a hierarchy of disability. There is a reluctance to imply that some disabled people are better or more worthy than others. Yet it seems to me inescapable that some forms of impairments are more limiting than others. Some disabled people are very restricted by their impairments, and others are not.

A precise ranking of impairment is of course very difficult, because it depends on subjective or cultural judgements as to how different factors are weighted: presence of pain, reduced life expectancy, visibility, mobility and other aspects would presumably be viewed differently by different people. It seems likely that, in general, disabled people come to terms with their own personal circumstances, while often thinking of other impairments as harder to deal with: the human capacity for accomodation and adaptation to adverse circumstances is extraordinary (Albrecht and Devlieger, 1999). Despite the reluctance to admit it, there are many instances of disabled people themselves adopting a hierachy of impairment (Deal, 2003).

None of these claims contradict two important points which disability studies has asserted strongly. First, non-disabled people generally perceive impairment to be far more negative and limiting than those who experience it directly (Young, 1997). Second, social barriers and social oppression are major factors in the lives of people with impairment, and for many disabled people cause more problems than their impairment. A key dimension of disability is the extent to which a society removes barriers and enables people to participate, regardless of their individual differences. The value of the social model tradition is in highlighting oppression and exclusion, issues which have been neglected in all previous research on disability. Yet impairment almost always plays some role in the lives of disabled people, even if social arrangements or cultural context minimises the exclusion or disadvantage.

As the Dutch research highlights, the interactional approach also makes space for an often neglected aspect of disablement: personal attitudes and motivation. It is not just the extent or nature of impairment, or the extent of the barriers and oppression which dictates the extent of disadvantage. For example, people with very similar impairments in the same society have different experiences, depending on their attitudes and reactions to their situation. Enabling disabled people to take a more positive approach and enhancing their self-esteem and self-confidence may sometimes transform their lives as much as providing better facilities or access to medical treatments. Joining a self-advocacy or disability rights group can change an individual's attitudes to themselves and their situation, enabling them to take control of their lives and become more effective.

The interactional approach also highlights the different ways in which the situation of disabled people can be improved. Traditional approaches to disability stress medical cure and rehabilitation. Social model approaches stress barrier removal and anti-discrimination legislation. For example, Michael Oliver has suggested that:

> the social model is not an attempt to deal with the personal restrictions of impairment but the social barriers of disability . . . [It is a] pragmatic attempt to identify and address issues that can be changed through collective action rather than medical or professional treatment.
>
> (Oliver, 1996: 38)

However, the reality is that disabled people are affected by physical, psychological and external problems. A theory which addresses only external barriers is an incomplete response to the challenge of disability. Substituting medical or professional treatment for social change and barrier removal is also unacceptable. Both approaches are needed.

An interactional approach allows for the different levels of experience, ranging from the medical, through the psychological, to the environmental, economic and political. Rather than dismissing individual interventions as reactionary and structural change as progressive, this approach allows each option to be discussed on its merits. An interactional approach would suggest there are many different factors which could be addressed to improve quality of life: coaching or therapy to improve self-esteem; medical intervention to restore functioning or reduce pain; aids and adaptations; barrier removal; anti-discrimination and attitudinal change; better benefits and services. Given the multiple and non-contradictory options for intervention, a debate is needed as to which approach is the most appropriate or cost-effective for different impairments or specific individuals. There can be no prior assumption that one approach is automatically preferable in all cases. The notion of *appropriate interventions* suggests that judgements about how to improve individual situations are complex, and should be based on evidence, not ideology. Cases such as limb-lengthening, cochlear implants and cosmetic surgery for children with Down syndrome illustrate the contested nature of these decisions. Evaluations of particular new technologies – for example, the Ibot wheelchairs which can negotiate steps and raise individuals to reach high and make eye contact – are also relevant. Such assistive technology overcomes architectural barriers: is investment in very expensive equipment a distraction from campaigning for universal design?

## Ubiquity of impairment

The interactional approach to understanding disability as a complex and multifactorial phenomenon necessitates coming to terms with impairment. Critiquing the social model, I argued that impairment was important to many disabled people, and had to be adequately theorised in any social theory of disability. Until now, only two alternatives have been offered: what Michael Oliver calls 'medical tragedy theory', and the denial or neglect of impairment within social model theory. Impairment is not the end of the world, tragic and pathological. But neither is it irrelevant, or just another difference. Many disabled people are unable to view impairment as neutral, as Michael Oliver and Bob Sapey concede in the second edition of *Social Work with Disabled People*:

> Some disabled people do experience the onset of impairments as a personal tragedy which, while not invalidating the argument that they are being excluded from a range of activities by a disabling environment, does mean it would be inappropriate to deny that impairment can be experienced in this way.
>
> (Oliver and Sapey, 1998: 26)

Instead of the polarised and one-dimensional accounts in both traditional research and disability studies, a nuanced attitude is needed, involving a fundamental ambivalence. Disability studies needs to capture the fact that impairment may not be neutral, but neither is it always all-defining and terrible.

One way of capturing the complexity of impairment is to view it as a *predicament*. *The Concise Oxford Dictionary* defines predicament as 'an unpleasant, trying or dangerous situation'. Although still negative, this does not have the inescapable emphasis of 'tragedy'. The notion of 'trying' perhaps captures the difficulties which many impairments present. They make life harder, although this hardship can be overcome. The added burdens of social oppression and social exclusion, which turn impairment into disadvantage, need to be removed: this seems to me very much the spirit of the original UPIAS approach to disability. Everything possible needs to be provided to make coping with impairment easier. But even with the removal of barriers and the provision of support, impairment will remain problematic for many disabled people.

For example, I have restricted growth. This is a very visible impairment, but is comparatively minor. The main effect in daily life is that many people stare at me. This is because the vast majority of people do not have restricted growth and are unfamiliar with people with restricted growth. For them, and particularly for children, dwarfs are fascinating. Education can reduce but will never eliminate this natural curiosity. Therefore, I will always be stared at. This is not pleasant, even if people are not actually hostile. I cannot escape the awareness of my abnormal embodiment, however much I am happy and successful as an individual. But I do not think these reactions can easily be explained away as oppression. They are a fact of life, like the vulnerability to back problems which is another dimension of my impairment. No amount of civil rights or social inclusion will entirely remove either of these dimensions of my predicament as a dwarf.

Similarly, many of the persistent environmental barriers discussed previously might better be theorised as predicaments. The predicament of impairment – the intrinsic difficulties of engaging with the world, the pains and sufferings and limitations of the body – mean that impairment is not neutral. It may bring insights and experiences which are positive, and for some these may even outweigh the disadvantages. But that does not mean that we should not try and minimise the number of people who are impaired, or the extent to which they are impaired.

It is not only impairment which is a predicament. For example, Zygmunt Bauman argues that 'The postmodern mind is reconciled to the idea that the messiness of the human predicament is here to stay. This is, in the broadest of outlines, what can be called postmodern wisdom' (Bauman, 1993: 245). Other aspects of embodiment – for example, the pains of menstruation or childbirth for women – could also be understood through the predicament concept, as could the inevitability and tragedy of death. To call something a predicament is to understand it as a difficulty, and as a challenge, and as something which we might want to minimise but which we cannot ultimately avoid. As Sebastiano Timpanaro suggests, 'physical ill . . . cannot be ascribed solely to bad social arrangements: it has its zone of autonomous and invincible reality' (Timpanaro, 1975: 20). But this is not to fall into the trap of regarding impairment as a tragedy or an identity-defining flaw.

Some people will object to what appears to be a negative approach to impairment. They should note that I am not denigrating disabled people, nor claiming that impairment makes disabled people second-class citizens or less worthy of support and respect. Disabled people are often inferior to non-disabled people in terms of health, function or ability, but they are not lesser in terms of moral worth, political equality or human rights. The suffering and happiness of disabled people matters just as much as that of non-disabled people.

If impairment truly was neutral – or beneficial – then we could have no objection to someone who deliberately impaired a child. If impairment was just another difference, then, as John Harris (1993; 2001) points out, there would be nothing wrong with painlessly altering a baby so they could no longer see, or could no longer hear, or had to use a wheelchair. Even if no suffering or pain was caused in the process, we would surely consider this irresponsible and immoral. Something would have been lost. The implication of this must be that impairment prevention should have an important role in social responses to disability. This does not undermine the worth or citizenship of existing disabled people. It suggests that because impairment causes predicaments and is limiting in various ways, we should take steps to prevent or mitigate it, where possible, as I will discuss in the second part of this book.

Furthermore, the connection to other embodiment predicaments underlines a commonplace observation which was made central in the work of Irving Zola (1989), and which has great significance for a post-social model approach to disability (see also Bickenbach et al., 1999). Impairment is a universal phenomenon, in the sense that every human being has limitations and vulnerabilities (Sutherland, 1981) and ultimately is mortal. Across the life span, everyone experiences impairment and limitation. Impairment is more likely to be acquired than congenital: ageing is particularly associated with increased levels of impairment. The ubiquity of impairment is underscored by the Human Genome Project which has shown that everyone has hundreds of mutations in their genome, many of which may predispose the individual to illness or impairment. In this sense, genetic diagnosis is toxic knowledge, which has the power to turn healthy people into pre-impaired people.

To claim that 'everyone is impaired' should not lead to any trivialising of impairment or the experience of disabled people. As I have stated previously, impairments differ in their impact. It is important to respect real differences – particularly the extent to which people are affected by suffering and restriction. At the extreme, as Alastair Macintyre argues, are very severely impaired people, 'such that they can never be more than passive members of the community, not recognizing, not speaking or not speaking intelligibly, suffering, but not acting' (1999: 127). It would be wrong to neglect the particular needs which arise from these different differences.

Not everyone is impaired all the time. Taking a life course view of impairment highlights the ways that impairment is manifested over time: disabled children grow up to be non-disabled adults, non-disabled people become impaired through accident or in old age. Impairments can be variable and episodic: sometimes people recover, and sometimes impairments worsen. The nature and meaning of impairment is not given in any one moment. Not all people with impairment have the same needs, or are disadvantaged to the same extent. Morever, different people experience different levels of social disadvantage or social exclusion, because society is geared to accommodate people with certain impairments, but not others. Everyone may be impaired, but not everyone is oppressed.

The benefits of regarding every human being as living with the predicament of impairment are that it forces us to pay attention to what we have in common; it counsels us to accept the inextricable limitation of life, rather than to deny or fight against it; it suggests the need to re-evaluate disabled people; it focuses attention on the social aspects of disability. For example, if everyone is impaired, why are certain impairments remedied or accepted, and others not? Why does impairment result in exclusion in some cases and not others? These processes and choices are largely social and structural and can be changed. In policy terms, a universal approach would use the range of human variation as the basis for universal design, and aim for justice in the distribution of resources and opportunities. Disabled people would not be expected to identify themselves as separate and incompetent, in order to qualify for provision.

## Conclusion

The complex reality of impairment suggests that equalising the situation for disabled people will necessarily be more complex and difficult than equalising the situation for women and other minorities. In the previous chapter, I argued that there were differences between disability, on the one hand, and race, gender and sexuality on the other, because disability was connected to intrinsic disadvantage. As Jerome Bickenbach *et al.* (1999) have argued, disabled people experience both restrictions of negative freedom – in the form of discrimination which prevents them achieving their potential – but also restrictions of positive freedom because they cannot participate freely in society. 'The denial of opportunities and resources is an issue, not of discrimination, but of distributive injustice – an unfair distribution of social resources and opportunities that results in limitations of participation in all areas of social life' (Bickenbach *et al.*,1999: 110).

Ending disablism – unfair discrimination against disabled people – will not solve all the problems of disabled people. Even if environments and transports were accessible and there was no unfair discrimination on the basis of disability, many disabled people would still be disadvantaged. For example, it is well known that some impairments generate extra costs – heating, equipment, diet (Smith *et al.*, 2005). Many disabled people require personal assistance or care. And while many disabled people could work just as productively as non-disabled people, once discrimination was fully removed, this does not apply to all disabled people. Some disabled people are unable to work a seven-hour day or a five-day week, due to fatigue. Some disabled people are unable to work at the intensity or productivity of non-disabled workers. Some disabled people are very limited in the types of tasks they are able to perform. And, of course, some disabled people are entirely unable to work.

This problem has been noted by several commentators. For example, Henley (2001) discusses the ways in which the emphasis on normalisation in policy towards people with learning difficulties in the 1980s led to the closing of day centres and other projects. In 1984 the King's Fund published *An Ordinary Working Life*, which stated that paid employment for all people with learning difficulties was an achievable aim (Henley, 2001: 940). While many more people with learning difficulties undoubtedly can work than were working at the time, it is unrealistic to suggest tht this is an option for all:

> The lesson to be learnt from the past is that the policy of pursuing total inclusion for all people with learning disabilities and encouraging the decimation of all forms of specialist service support in the process has, in practice, proved to be fundamentally flawed.
>
> (Henley, 2001: 946)

Paul Abberley also notes that 'even in a society which did make profound, genuine attempts, well supported by a financial provision, to integrate profoundly impaired people into the world of work, some would be excluded' (Abberley, 2001: 131). Paul Hunt (1966) also challenged the focus on work, arguing that disabled people outside the labour market contributed to society in different ways, not least by challenging utilitarian values.

Analysing the Disability Discrimination Act, Gooding argues that more is required than treating everyone the same (Gooding, 2000: 536). Society's failure to meet the needs of disabled people cannot be accounted for simply by the concept of disablism. The strategy of promoting employment, while very desirable, will also leave a residuum of unemployed and unemployable disabled people. Disability includes intrinsic limitation and disadvantage. Societies will need to address this, by making additional investment to equalise the situation between disabled and non-disabled people – not just equal opportunities, but redistribution.

While disability studies and disability rights movements have criticised individual and medical approaches to disability, the focus on civil rights still implies a liberal solution to the disability problem (Russell, 2002). Anti-discrimination law and independent living solutions seem to suggest that the market will provide, if only disabled people are enabled to exercise choices free of unfair discrimination. But market approaches often restrict, rather than increase, choice to disabled people (Williams, 1983; Wilson *et al.*, 2000). An individual, market-based solution, by failing to acknowledge persistant inequalities in physical and mental capacities, cannot liberate all disabled people.

Human beings are not all the same, and do not all have the same capabilities and limitations. Need is variable, and disabled people are among those who need more from others and from their society. Alastair Macintyre begins to explore the political implications of this reality:

> a form of political society in which it is taken for granted that disability and dependence on others are something that all of us experience at certain times in our lives and this to unpredictable degrees, and that consequently our interest in how the needs of the disabled are adequately voiced and met is not a special interest, the interest of one particular group rather than of others, but rather the interest of the whole political society, an interest that is integral to their conception of their common good.
>
> (Macintyre, 1999: 130)

This seems as radical as, and more adequate than, a social model denial of the persistance of impairment as a factor in creating disadvantage. Impairment is not usually a matter of individual responsibility: it arises from the random effect of genes or disease, or the socially created costs of work, warfare, poverty, or from the natural effects of the ageing process. If disabled people have equal moral worth to non-disabled people – and are viewed politically as equal citizens – then justice demands social arrangements which compensate for both the natural lottery and socially caused injury. Creating a level playing field is not enough: redistribution is required to promote true social inclusion.

# Chapter 5

# Labels and badges

## The politics of disability identity

## Introduction

There is a strong consensus in the disability studies literature that the disability movement has been a very positive force, both in the collective ability to lever political change and in the benefits to individual participants (Driedger, 1989; Gilson *et al.*, 1997; Charlton, 1998; Branfield, 1999) – 'A confident, positive disability identity within a broad, inclusive disability community has emerged. The benefit to disabled people to determine and relate their own stories is increasingly evident' (Gilson *et al.*, 1997: 16).

Many disability studies researchers – including myself – have been active in, or have emerged out of, the disability rights struggle. The principle of emancipatory research (Mercer, 2002) suggests that disability studies should be accountable to the priorities and organisations of disabled people. Perhaps this very closeness leads to an unquestioning acceptance of the benefits of political affiliation and an affirmatory reading of disability identity politics.

For example, Jane Campbell and Michael Oliver's social history of the disability movement gives a largely positive account of the political developments of the 1970s and 1980s. The growth of political consciousness and collective organisation was welcomed by many contributors, particularly because it built the self-esteem of individual participants. The social model came as an immense liberation (Campbell and Oliver, 1996: 117). Conscientisation (Freire, 1972) through disability rights analysis changes a person's self-conception. As James Charlton suggests,

> The critical consciousness that emerges from this position may lead some people to adopt the disability activist subject position which can involve street level political action or challenging and transforming the organisations for the disabled to become organisations of disabled people and so on. In this sense, to name disability as social oppression is not the defeated wailings of victims, but the clarion call of social change agents.
>
> (Charlton, 1998: 192)

One example of this mobilisation is provided by the Deaf community. During the 1970s, Deaf people began organising as a social movement, challenging the idea that they were impaired, and defining themselves increasingly as a linguistic minority, using the model of ethnicity. In this period, slogans such as Deaf Pride and Deaf Power became popular. One of the culminations of this new Deaf identity and political consciousness came with the successful 1988 Deaf President Now protest at Gallaudet University. After the appointment of a hearing president at this university for the Deaf, students exploded into political action, closing down the college in order to demand that the Board of Trustees appoint the first deaf president in the school's history. As two analysts commented:

> The transformation involved deaf persons: (a) identifying themselves as members of a community sharing common values and traits (e.g. sign language) and (b) evaluating the group and its values and traits in a positive light. Ironically, as a group's members come to value themselves after a long period of self deprecation, the consciousness-raising can lead to anger, resentment, and political action over the perceived injustices.
>
> (Rose and Kiger, 1995: 522)

The same anger can be seen in the direct action of disabled people in many countries of the world (which is well documented in Charlton, 1998). John Swain and Sally French (2000) have even suggested a new conception of disability, which they term an affirmation model. This combines a focus on the political benefits of identifying with a collectivity, but also a redefinition of the nature of impairment. For example, impairment is seen to bring benefits such as being able to escape role restrictions and social expectations, the possibility of empathy with others and better relationships:

> In affirming a positive identity of being impaired, disabled people are actively repudiating the dominant value of normality. The changes for individuals are not just a transforming of consciousness as to the meaning of 'disability', but an assertion of the value and validity of life as a person with an impairment.
>
> (Swain and French, 2000: 578)

For Swain and French, the role of disability culture – for example, disability arts cabarets – is central to this process. Campbell and Oliver's contributors also stress the role of direct action and other collective forms of political process, which give disabled people the feelings of power and validation, and provide a symbolic challenge to an oppressive and exclusionary society. The implication of these studies is to suggest that the growth of disability politics has created new social forms, and new possibilities for individual affiliation and identity. Bill Hughes *et al.*, reviewing the issues for young disabled people in contemporary culture, claim that 'The growth of disability pride suggests that disabled people do not want to be other than they are. They are not rejecting disability as an identity or trying to escape the biological realities of impairment' (Hughes *et al.*, 2005: 7).

My worry with this suggestion is that it implies that disability identity is a given, and that impairment will automatically define personal identity. Instead, I would claim that disability politics offers new options for individuals to think about both their impairment, and their position in society. Following Ian Hacking (1986), I suggest that the rise of disability politics has created a new category, a new way of affiliating and identifying, which did not exist before.

Some scholars and activists have actively tried to develop the notion of a disability identity, suggesting that it is appropriate to talk in terms of disability culture, and affirming an ethnic conception of disability identity. Susan Peters (2000) argues that there is a disability culture just as there is a Deaf culture. She points to a common language, a shared historical lineage, cohesive social community, and political solidarity. For her, the Independent Living community in Berkeley was the equivalent of Martha's Vineyard for Deaf people. Peters quotes Carol Gill, 'I believe very firmly in disabled culture – and if we don't have one we should. We need it to survive as an oppressed minority, both physically and emotionally' (Peters, 2000: 584). In the same vein, Fran Branfield has called for a separatist approach to disability research (Branfield, 1998, 1999).

In passing, I note that an interesting feature of the work on disability as a political identity is that it shows that the social barriers approach which is the defining characteristic of the UK social model actually overlaps with, or subsumes, a minority group conception. A social barriers approach does not define a particular group who are to benefit from barrier removal; it implicitly refuses to identify people with impairments as a distinct group. But in the practices of the disability movement, clearly a group emerges of people with impairment who are campaigning both for removal of barriers, and for better provision for their minority. In other words, rather than seeing a major distinction between US and UK strategies, there is overlap between minority group and barriers theory. US approaches are framed in terms of the minority group approach, but contain an emphasis on social barriers; UK approaches are framed in terms of the barriers approach, but contain a strong element of minority group conception. For example, Michael Oliver's discussion of disability identity suggests that it comprises three elements: having an impairment; experiencing externally imposed restrictions; self-identification as a disabled person (Oliver, 1996: 5).

In this chapter I will challenge some of the taken-for-granted assumptions about the benefits of disability identity. First, I will explore the tension between labels and badges. Then I will critically evaluate the extent to which disabled people do identify politically, and the representativeness of the disability movement. Next I will explore some of the problems with identity politics, particularly in the case of disability, before concluding with an alternative account of emancipatory politics, drawn from the work of Nancy Fraser.

## Labels and badges

It is paradoxical that the identification of people with impairment as members of a disabled collective is generally viewed positively, whereas the ascription of group membership – in the form of labelling – is generally viewed negatively in the disability community. Deconstruction of these processes – the difference between a badge and a label – is important in understanding the complexity of identification.

In the previous chapter, I showed how scepticism about medical categories is often signalled with scare quotes. Within the field of learning difficulties, the influence of normalisation has led to an opposition to form of medical or psychological diagnosis or labelling (Gillman *et al.*, 2000; Chappell *et al.*, 2001). Opposition to labelling arises from an awareness of the stigma which can be a consequence of particular labels or diagnoses. When someone is given a label – for example of learning disability or mental illness – this may trigger other negative associations. The phenomenon of 'identity spread' means that the person's individuality – not only their personality, but also other aspects of their identity such as gender, sexuality and ethnicity – can be ignored, as the impairment label becomes the most prominent and relevant feature of their lives, dominating interactions.

There are several reasons to qualify the opposition to labelling. Barbara Riddick (2000) points out that stigma can happen even without labelling. In theory at least, labelling can happen without stigma. Moreover, for some groups, diagnosis is a very important and valuable process. My colleague Steve Macdonald researches the experiences of people diagnosed as dyslexic. He argues strongly that diagnosis is valued by his respondents, because it enables them to see themselves not as intellectually limited, but as having a particular brain difference. Moreover, a diagnosis enables people with dyslexia to get the computer technology and educational support they need to survive in school and university. Similarly, Fox and Kim (2004) argue that people with what they call 'emerging disabilities' – which are often invisible – are struggling to achieve medical acceptance. Such individuals positively welcome a label:

> While many interest groups of persons with disabilities are highly vocal in their desire to disconnect their disability from medical diagnosis and treatment, groups of persons with disabilities perceived as emerging stage their early battles for this very turf, hoping that medical acceptance will lead to greater social acceptance.
>
> (Fox and Kim, 2004: 334)

Diagnosis for people with hidden impairments gives credibility to their difference, may lead to effective medical or educational support, and also gives protection under anti-discrimination legislation such as the Americans with Disabilities Act.

Understanding that an impairment is real, and may have a biological basis, has been liberating for families affected by autism: in previous generations, parents were blamed for having emotionally deprived their children. But Hodge (2005) reflects on ambivalence about the process of diagnosis in the case of autistic spectrum disorders. Diagnosis can lead to better understanding of the problem and access to appropriate support mechanisms: resource allocation is label-led. But a diagnosis can also be disempowering for parents, causing them to fear for the future. There is also a danger of seeing the label, not the individual child. Equally, minimising the extent to which autism is an impairment – seeing it simply as 'an alternative way of being' could be a denial of the pervasive and devestating impact of autism on both the child and the family.

Labelling is a complex and paradoxical process (Brown, 1995; Shakespeare and Erickson, 2000). For example, Clarke *et al.* (2005) points out the contradiction between defining an individual with impairment as normal within family and community, but at the same time needing to identify them as abnormal to get services and benefits. A similar paradox surrounds political identification as disabled, as I will discuss below: people who would oppose labelling and reject medical diagnoses are nevertheless willing to identify politically as disabled and accept a badge or banner. Yet, as I show, many people with impairments do not want to identify either as impaired (with a label) or disabled (with a badge): they want to be seen as ordinary members of society, free of limitation or classification.

## Identification as disabled

Notwithstanding the positive disability studies assessment of the disability movement, there are important questions about the extent to which people with impairment identify with the disability movement, or indeed as people with impairment. Despite the visibility of disability rights protest, it has always been a minority activity for disabled people. For example, the Direct Action Network may be very vocal, but it now appears to number less than 100 people, with approximately 30 attending recent demonstrations. Even at the height of disability protest, approximately 2,000 disabled people joined the 1988 Elephant and Castle demonstration (Campbell and Oliver, 1996). Given that there are more than six million disabled people in Britain, this represents a small proportion of the potential support.

Of course, lack of activism does not necessarily imply lack of affiliation to the values or demands of the disability rights movement. Other liberation movements – such as the women's movement and the lesbian and gay movement – have never mobilised a significant proportion of their communities. Moroever, due to transport barriers and mobility and income restrictions, it is harder for disabled people to mobilise. Therefore it is important to look to other research to understand the extent to which disabled people view themselves as part of a larger minority group. *Disabled for Life?*, a research project undertaken by the Department for Work and Pensions in 2003 found that 52 per cent of Disability Discrimination Act (DDA) defined disabled people did not define themselves as disabled people: young people were particularly likely to reject this identification. However, this might indicate a reluctance to identify with a stigmatised social label, and an ignorance of the social model redefinition of disability. A 2002 survey of 200 disabled people conducted by the British Council of Disabled People found that only 3 per cent of them had heard of the social model (Rickell, 2006).

Bob Sapey, John Stuart and Glenis Donaldson (2005) conducted research in north-west England to explore reasons for the increase in use of wheelchairs, and to investigate perceptions of disability: over 1,000 responded to their survey. Nearly 80 per cent of respondents agreed that wheelchairs can be liberating for disabled people. Forty-eight per cent of people agreed that the environment around them made it hard for them to do many things they wanted to do in their wheelchair. But 80 per cent of people also agreed that their illness or condition stopped them doing many things they wanted to do – which is far from a social model position. The authors of the study claim that the findings are consistent with the social model of disability, and show that social model analysis is relevant to lived experience. This appears to me to be a rather selective reading of the data, which suggests that both impairment and environment are implicated in the experience of disability, supporting the interactional conception of disability which was proposed in the previous chapter.

Turning to qualitative research, several studies challenge a simplistic social model identification. For example, in Kelly's research with young people with autism, respondents' experiences and affiliations could not straightforwardly be subsumed under the social model:

> A social model of disability that focuses on oppressive barriers in society does not fully account for the experiences of children involved in this study. Findings reveal their experiences and feelings about impairment. Impairment and disability were particularly significant experiences for some children and not so important for others. For some children, experiences of impairment (such as not being able to understand or desiring to be able to walk) were just as important as disabling structures in society. For others, experience of disabling barriers in society (such as adult surveillance or exclusions from social opportunities) were more salient than their experience of impairment.
>
> (Kelly, 2005: 271)

Jane Andrews's research with disabled volunteers found that neither a medical model nor a social model approach satisfactorily explained her data:

> In particular, the volunteers interviewed during the pre-field and pilot stages of the study continually expressed frustration with the medically derived limitations placed upon them as individuals living with various illnesses and impairments. Such limitations appeared to them to be more restrictive than any socially constructed barriers encountered during the normal day-to-day routines of volunteering.
>
> (Andrews, 2005: 203)

Nick Watson conducted an in-depth qualitative study with twenty-eight disabled people in Scotland. Despite daily experiences of oppressive practices, only three of the participants incorporated disability within their identity. Instead, they normalised their experience of physical limitation. They were all able to describe experiences of discrimination. But they rejected a political identity as disabled people:

> Being disabled, for many of these informants, is not about celebrating difference or diversity, pride in their identity is not formed through the individuals labelling themselves as different, as disabled, but it is about defining disability in their own terms, under their own terms of reference.
>
> (Watson, 2002: 521)

Their wish was to assimilate with the mainstream and negate a demeaning difference. We found a similar response when we did research with young disabled people in the late 1990s: while they could identify exclusionary processes and lack of access as problems, their goal to was to be part of the mainstream youth culture, not to identify themselves as disabled (Priestley *et al*., 1999).

The implication of early disability activism that people with impairments were oppressed and that salvation lay in collective identification and mobilisation has proved over-optimistic: only a tiny proportion of people with impairments have ever signed up to the radical campaign, and many have actively disowned it. Many people do not want to see themselves as disabled, either in terms of the medical model or the social model. They downplay the significance of their impairments. But neither do they see themselves as part of the disability movement, nor do they identify with a political conception of disability. They see themselves as 'really normal', refusing to allow disability to dominate their lives. Recognising this, the UK Disability Rights Commission no longer use the term disabled people: instead, they refer to 'people who have rights under the Disability Discrimination Act' (Fletcher, 2006). The refusal to define oneself by impairment or disability has sometimes been seen as 'internalised oppression' or 'false consciousness' by radicals in the disability movement. Yet this attitude can itself be patronising and oppressive. After all, the denial of disability is implicitly based on the rejection of the idea of an exclusive 'normality', and a refusal to be categorised. This approach may be rather individualist, and may overlook the problems of discrimination and prejudice. But surely it is a legitimate alternative to a minority group approach.

## Is the disability movement representative?

Above, I argued that the majority of disabled people do not identify themselves with the social model or in terms of a disability identity. A related issue is the extent to which the disability rights movement is representative of the disabled population as a whole. The disability movement in many countries is dominated by a somewhat restricted section of the impaired population. For example, in western countries, approximately half of all people with impairments are over the age of 50. Yet most activists enter the movement at a much younger age, and older people who have impairments neither make up a significant proportion of the movement, nor are likely to identify with a civil rights perspective.

Again, there have been persistent questions about the role and involvement of particular impairment groups. For example, people with learning difficulties may have been excluded because their particular access and language issues have not been properly understood, or because they have not been welcomed, or because social model theory has not effectively incorporated intellectual impairments (Chappell, 1998; Chappell *et al.*, 2001). Some disabled people have sought to bolster their own status as people with physical impairments at the expense of those with intellectual impairments. Another example is the Deaf community, who have resisted identification with the mainstream disability movement. Often this is because Deaf people see themselves as a linguistic minority, not as people defined by a medical condition: of course, some disabled people themselves have rejected a medical identity, so perhaps the problem is less one of definition, and more about separate cultures (Corker, 1998). More of a problem is that dominant disability rights demands – such as inclusive education for all disabled children – are rejected by Deaf communities who want their children separately educated via the medium of sign language. Deaf politics found it easier to adopt a straightforward identity politics model, as the movements for Deaf Pride and Deaf Power demonstrate. Rose and Kiger (1995) use the social psychologist Henri Tajfel (1978) to explore this process of a hitherto excluded community acquiring a 'voice' through social action to enhance the interests of a minority group, which comes to see itself as oppressed minority. To bolster their self-image, a group exaggerates and values its members' distinctiveness. A sense of of injustice and resistance leads to increased identification with the group, which also promotes the self-esteem of its members.

Aside from differences of impairment and age, other social cleavages are also evident in disability politics, which has failed to account for the diversity of identity (Vernon, 1996, 1999). Feminists have often criticised the disability movement for sexism and the exclusion of women's issues. Minority ethnic communities have sometimes felt ignored by disability groups dominated by the majority population. Lesbian and gay disabled people have experienced homophobia, or have felt unwelcome in disability organisations which have taken on radical disabled perspectives, but may be very conventional in terms of sexual politics. Finally, access to economic and social power is a strong determinant of the life-experience of disabled people in general, and also influences involvement in disability politics: many leaders of the movement have come from privileged socio-economic contexts. Nor, as Gary Albrecht suggests, have civil rights approaches benefited poorer disabled people:

> The problem with this approach is that it accomplishes little or nothing for poor and marginal Americans. Grass roots activism is confined principally to the educated middle class who are savvy about lobbying. The poor and

marginal Americans do not represent themselves well and are not effectively represented by liberals. The result is that those most in need of services are least likely to receive help, especially in economic hard times.

(Albrecht, 1992: 300)

If the disability movement (and disability studies) has not been fully represen-tative of the variety of disabled people's experiences, then perhaps this suggests another reason for the inadequacies of the social model approach. The activists of UPIAS were predominantly people with physical impairments, mainly wheelchair users. Their conceptualisation of disability may have reflected the specificity of their own experience. For example, people with spinal cord injury, once stabilised, do not suffer degenerating chronic illness. There may be vulnerability to pressure sores or urinary infections, but these may seem like management and hygiene issues. To a wheelchair user, their health may not be the problem, whereas the lack of physical access and the prejudices of employers and professionals might well be. In other words, the social model possibly works from the perspective of someone with a stable physical impairment. But had the original UPIAS ideological discussions included people with mental health issues, people with learning difficulties, or even people whose physical impairments involved more intrinsic pain and suffering, then perhaps a richer and more complex understanding of the nature of disability might have resulted.

## Challenges to disability identity

Disability identity politics has been very powerful, but also contradictory and incoherent. This may derive from the heterogeneity of disabled people's experience. As Bickenbach *et al.* note, the analogy between racial minorities and disabled people breaks down at many important points:

> Not only are the social responses to different forms of mental and physical impairments vastly different, from the other direction there is almost no commonality of experience, or feelings of solidarity, between people with diverse disabilities. There is no unifying culture, language or set of experiences; people with disabilities are not homogenous, nor is there much prospect for transdisability solidarity.

(Bickenbach *et al.*, 1999: 1181)

A pure barriers approach does not specify a group of subjects who could adopt a political identity as disabled. But, equally, the basis of disabled identity could not be located in impairment. The social model was based on the irrelevance of impairment to the definition of disability. Moreover, impairment is negatively valued socially. Slogans such as 'glad to be gay', 'black is beautiful' do not have an equivalent in the disability movement. Therefore the basis of identity had to be found in shared resistance to oppression, similar to the feminist slogan 'sisterhood is powerful'. Without a basis in impairment, disability identity becomes voluntaristic and difficult to define or police. Disabled people become classed as the category of people who identify as having experienced disability oppression. For example, Simi Linton suggests that 'The question of who "qualifies" as disabled is as answerable or as confounding as questions about any identity status. One simple response might be that you are disabled if you say you are' (Linton, 1998: 12).

The UK-based organisation Disability Awareness in Action similarly states that 'DAA's work is driven by an inclusive view of the disabled community – defined quite simply as those who choose to identify as disabled' (Disability Awareness in Action, n.d.,). However, this approach would include some people who happen to like the idea of being members of a disabled minority group, but in objective terms are not oppressed in any way. It would also exclude some people who may objectively experience oppression, but subjectively refuse to identify themselves as oppressed. It may also include people who may experience forms of social exclusion based on physical difference, but would not traditionally be seen as disabled. For example, one writer asks whether a fat woman can call herself disabled:

> Many fat people suffer poor self-esteem, we grow up fearing our own bodies in shame, public ridicule and social ostracism, and the cultural fear and hatred of us can ruin our lives. I believe that self-defining as 'disabled' enables us to take ourselves seriously and demand that others do also.
>
> (Cooper, 1997: 33)

In developing a social model approach to fatness, Cooper shows how defining disability in terms of social barriers or social oppression, rather than a biological impairment, opens up the category to a range of other social excluded or devalued groups: what about anorexic women (Tierney, 2001)? If 'disabled people' emerge as a result of individual political action or group affiliation, it becomes an artificial, contingent and ultimately unsatisfactory grouping.

A deeper set of challenges question the form that disability identity takes, particularly the ethnic or cultural conception of disability. For example, Humphrey (1999; 2000) has challenged the separatism of identity-based approaches. Researching disability identity in the context of a trades union disability network, she argues that self-definition is problematic, because self-defined people may be suspected of not really being disabled. Failure to discuss impairment benefits those with visible impairments, and makes it harder to discuss impairment-related needs:

> [T]he social model as operationised within the UNISON group has both reified the disability identity and reduced it to particular kinds of impairments – physical, immutable, tangible and 'severe' ones – in a way which can deter many people from adopting a disabled identity and participating in a disability community.
>
> (Humphrey, 2000: 69)

Humphrey also criticises the opposition of disabled to non-disabled people which results from an exclusive version of disability identity:

> In terms of identity, this leaves no scope to deal adequately with those who cross-over between disabled and non-disabled worlds, or those who inhabit a liminal space. In terms of politics, it lends itself to a separatism which closes off many doors to coalition and transformation.
>
> (Humphrey, 2000: 81)

The notion of disability identity raises particular problems. But any resort to identity politics is problematic. The logic of identity politics can prove counter-productive. At one level, this arises from the inexhaustible number of possible identities. Lennard Davis argues that identity politics is self-defeating, because ultimately everyone has an identity. 'The list of identities will only grow larger, tied to an ever expanding idea of inclusiveness. After all, when all identities are finally included, there will be no identity' (Davis, 2002: 88). As Phil Lee argues, socially constructed identities are 'contestable and subject to change; sub- and splinter groups emerge, as different aspects of the identity are prioritized' (Lee, 2002: 151).

But a more significant problem with a minority group approach to disability was first identified by Helen Liggett (1988) and draws on Foucauldian ideas. Disability politics, by its very nature, often rests on a fairly unreflexive acceptance of the disabled/non-disabled distinction. Disabled people are seen as those who identify as such. Disabled leadership is seen as vital. But Liggett argues:

> From an interpretative point of view the minority group approach is double edged because it means enlarging the discursive practices which participate in the constitution of disability . . . [I]n order to participate in their own management disabled people have had to participate as disabled. Even among the politically active, the price of being heard is understanding that it is the disabled who are speaking.
>
> (Liggett, 1988: 271ff.)

This relates to what Denise Riley has called 'the dangerous intimacy between subjectification and subjection' (Riley, 1988: 17). A minority group approach demands a dichotomy between disabled and non-disabled people, reinforcing differentness, rather than promoting assimilation. As Galvin argues,

> By claiming an identity which has been created though the processes of hierachical differentiation and exclusion, subjugated peoples reinforce their own oppression and restrict their hopes to the belief that they can demonstrate how positive it is to be identified as such.
>
> (Galvin, 2003: 682)

To be an activist – whether as a gay person, or a woman, or a disabled person – is to make the label into a badge, to make the ghetto into a oppositional culture. Yet what about those, like the disabled people cited earlier, who wish to be ordinary, not different? Post-structuralists such as Diane Fuss (1989) argue that an essentialist theory of identity, however attractive, is ultimately not a secure foundation for politics.

*badge vs label* (handwritten margin note)

However, there is potentially a higher price to adopting the disability label than just to highlight separateness and difference. A more serious problem, within the disability context, is that building an identity around oppression leads the minority group into taking up a victim position. In this sense, a social model of disability can be as negative as a medical model of disability. Whereas the latter sees disabled people as victims of their flawed bodies or brains, the former sees disabled people as prisoners of an oppressive and excluding society. In both versions, the agency of disabled people is denied and the scope for positive engagement with either impairment or society is diminished.

Building identity on victimhood leads to the recital of a litany of oppression and woe. For example, the editors of the revised edition of the seminal *Disabling Barriers – Enabling Environments* claim that in the ten years since the first edition, nothing has changed. 'Despite major changes in legislation, for instance, the dominant picture remains one of discrimination, prejudice, injustice and poverty, often rationalised on the grounds of supposed progress for disabled people' (Swain *et al.*, 2004: 1).

The activist and critic Paul Darke makes a similar but more extreme claim in a recent interview:

> On the surface, things are much better with many more opportunities than ever before. But underneath, things are actually much worse in the sense that even though we now have equality per se, legislation, access, whatever, 99 per cent of disabled people are being aborted or terminated or institutionalised or segregated. That's the reality for most disabled people.
>
> (Darke, 2004: 15)

Darke's claim is more rhetorical and has no basis in fact, but both statements paint a similarly negative picture. This way of thinking serves to obscure the progress which has been made over recent decades, often due to the political mobilisation of disabled people themselves. It is true that disabled people continue to do less well than the majority of society, and there is much to be done to ensure equality and inclusion. But attitudes to disabled people are slowly changing; the Disability Discrimination Act has mandated major access removal; more disabled people are entering employment; for people with learning difficulties, the Government's *Valuing People* paper (Department of Health, 2001), drafted with the participation of people with learning difficulties themselves, has put the principles of rights, independence, choice and inclusion at the centre of policy. Denying progress is as misguided as overlooking problems. The consequence of taking up a victim position and of exaggerating the differences and the polarity between the minority group and the mainstream is that politics can become more extreme, separatist, vanguardist and aggressive. The politics of coalition (Lee, 2002: 158) becomes less likely.

The victim position can be reassuring for individuals. It explains that any problems they might encounter, or failure they experience, has resulted from oppression, not from any fault of their own. It gives an excuse for not trying, because all efforts are doomed, and all change is illusory. The victim position also makes the success of other people who seemingly share your status very threatening. If some disabled people have achieved their goals, or have managed to be successful in a disabling society, then this undermines the victimhood analysis. For this reason, it becomes important to disown or condemn the 'tall poppies' who have succeeded.

Underlying identity politics, the social model can play an important psychological role for disabled people. It is a powerful way of denying both the relevance and the negativity of impairment. Activists can maintain that their problems are not due to their deficits of body or mind, but to the society in which they live. By combining with others who share this belief, their own self-image is reinforced, and they can achieve solidarity and self-respect. The social model became ideologically dominant precisely because it moved away from the individual and the personal and the psychological. This may explain how difficult it has been for social model perspectives to engage with the question of impairment: how could an identity-sustaining theory include what had been disavowed?

At the heart of the social model approach to disability is a kind of denial. Social model theory enables disabled people to deny the relevance of their impaired bodies or brains, and seek equality with non-disabled people on the basis of similarity. What divides disabled from non-disabled people, in this formulation, is the imposition of social oppression and social exclusion. Moreover, the identity politics which is fuelled by this ideology paradoxically depends on strengthening the coherence and separateness of the disability group. Disabled people are contrasted with non-disabled people. Non-disabled people and the non-disabled world are increasingly seen as oppressive and hostile. Those who claim to help disabled people – professionals, charities, governments – are rejected. A strong political identity, which should be a means to an end, has become an end in itself. Rather than looking outward, the disability movement has often turned inwards. Rather than building bridges with other groups or seeking the integration of its members within society, the vanguard of the disability movement has often been separatist, promoting a notion of 'us' disabled people against 'them' non-disabled oppressors (Holdsworth, 1993; Branfield, 1998, 1999). For disability activists this has been powerful and motivating, but as the basis for disability politics it has been counterproductive.

## Post-identity politics

Nancy Fraser (1995) has argued that radical social movements often combine a challenge to socio-economic injustice with a challenge to cultural injustice. She distinguishes between the politics of redistribution and the politics of recognition. What she calls 'bivalent collectivities' 'suffer both socioeconomic maldistribution and cultural misrecognition in forms where neither of these injustices is an indirect effect of the other, but where both are primary and co-original': in these cases, remedies for the two injustices may pull in different directions. She calls for transformational remedies – which deconstruct groupings and promote solidarity – rather than affirmative remedies, which leave deep structures intact and may even stigmatise the disadvantaged class. She also recognises that the politics of recognition can have negative effects, forcing individuals to conform to group culture and discouraging debate. 'The overall effect is to impose a single, drastically simplified group identity which denies the complexity of people's lives, the multiplicity of their identifications and the cross pulls of their various affiliations' (Fraser, 1995: 112).

For her, this version of identity politics can become repressive, intolerant and conformist, all adjectives which might be applied to the radical disability rights movement, which has encouraged exactly the separatism and group enclaves which Fraser fears.

The alternative which Fraser proposes is to seek recognition, not as a member of a disadvantaged group, but in terms of individual status. She suggests that 'To view recognition as a matter of status means examining institutionalised patterns of cultural value for their effects on the relative standing of social actors' (Fraser, 1995: 113). Rather than valorising group specificity and promoting essentialism, her social status approach to recognition may lead to a 'non-identitarian politics' in which 'Redressing misrecognition now means changing social institutions – or, more specifically, changing the interaction-regulating values that impede parity of recognition at all relevant institutional sites' (Fraser, 1995: 115).

While supportive of Fraser's approach, Berthe Danermark and L.C. Gellerstedt (2004) criticise Fraser for her lack of focus on face-to-face encounters. Like several other recent disability theorists, they look to the work of Axel Honneth (1995) to combine the different levels of misrecognition and injustice. Drawing on Mead and Hegel, Honneth looks at individual, social and cultural dimensions:

> This implies that injustices to disabled people can be understood neither as generated by solely cultural mechanisms (cultural reductionism) nor by socio-economic mechanisms (economic reductionism) nor by biological mechanisms (biological reductionism). In sum, only by taking different levels, mechanisms and contexts into account, can disability as a phenomenon be analytically approached.
>
> (Danermark and Gellerstedt, 2004: 350)

These different approaches may offer elements in a post-identity, post-social model disability politics. Such a re-conception is necessary to offer an alternative to the prison of identity politics, which leads to the politics of victimhood and the celebration of failure. Many disabled people will prefer to seek what they have in common with non-disabled people, promoting inclusion and equal status, not separatism. The goal of disability politics should be to make impairment and disability irrelevant wherever possible, not to seek out and celebrate a separatist notion of disability pride based on an ethnic conception of disability identity.

# Part II

# Disability and bioethics

# Chapter 6

# Questioning prenatal diagnosis

This chapter explores disability rights arguments about prenatal diagnosis (PND), challenging the basis on which objections have been expressed by activists and academics. However, I should state at the outset that my reluctance to accept certain arguments from disability rights critics of prenatal diagnosis does not entail support for prenatal diagnosis as it is currently practised. Nor do my arguments in this chapter imply acceptance of the positions of bioethicists such as John Harris (1985, 1992) or Peter Singer (1993). These utilitarian philosophers have argued strongly for screening, and even challenged opposition to infanticide in certain situations (Kuhse and Singer, 1985; Singer, 1993). Elsewhere, my colleague Simo Vehmas (2003a, 2003b, 2004) has developed a strong and well-argued philosophical critique of the assumptions and arguments about disability in this mainstream bioethical literature. While elsewhere I have tried to criticise both genetic practices and discourses about genetics and disability (Shakespeare 1995a, 1998, 1999a, 2005a), in this chapter I continue the revisionist work established earlier in this volume by critically analysing the basis of the disability rights critique.

## Is prenatal diagnosis eugenic?

Within the disability rights movement, there has been considerable concern about the scientific and societal enthusiasm for genetic research in contemporary western societies (Shakespeare, 1995; Asch, 2001; Goggin and Newell, 2005; Rock, 1996; Saxton, 2000). Disabled activists and authors have been prominent among those opposing developments in human genetics and reproductive medicine. But the critical and cautionary voices of disabled people have been largely absent from the policy and media debate about the impact of antenatal diagnosis on society. Looking at disability rights objections to antenatal diagnosis and selective termination, there are two linked themes: a powerful narrative about eugenics, and a claim about discrimination. In this and the succeeding section I will discuss these claims, and show why I believe that they cannot entirely be sustained.

The eugenic narrative suggests that new genetic technologies combine twenty-first century science with early twentieth century eugenic ideology. Particularly in activist literature, genetics becomes a coherent and consistent plot to eliminate disabled people. For example, a bioethics supplement of the international disability rights newsletter *Disability Awareness in Action* talked about disabled people as 'the target group for a "search and destroy" mission, both before and after birth, incorporating highly effective technologies' (Disability Awareness in Action, 1997: 1).

At about the same time as this was published, the International Centre for Life was being built in Newcastle, UK. This is a 'science village', funded by the Millennium Commission and the Wellcome Trust, where the public can visit an interactive science education centre on the same site as the University of Newcastle Institute of Human Genetics and other biomedical enterprises. Local activists of the disabled people's Direct Action Network carried out a demonstration at the building in 1997, using the slogan 'No Nazi Eugenics!' and Disability Action North East handed out a leaflet on 11 March 1998 which used phrases such as: 'eugenic agenda', 'Nazi-style programme of the Geneticists', '"virtual eugenics" theme park', and suggested that 'Geneticists desperately want to exploit disabled people . . . so they can achieve even greater power within the ranks of the medical empire and over society at large.'

When I was appointed to develop a bioethics and science engagement project on the same site, many disability rights activists condemned my decision to work with people they saw as the enemy. The equation of geneticists with Nazis is a frequent feature of critiques of this kind – 'Disabled people know only too well they are not welcomed in society, but the active promotion of abortion on the grounds of disability and determining that euthanasia is a viable proposition for the disabled foetus/child – is fascism' (Rock, 1996: 124).

No discussion of genetics should ignore the historical experience of Nazi euthanasia and eugenics. It is an important starting point for contemporary evaluations. For example, many have raised the spectre of Nazi eugenics as a reminder of what can go wrong with attempts to improve the health of the population (Bailey 1996: 144). This seems legitimate. It should be remembered that eugenic ideas were both common and widely supported in Europe and North America prior to 1945 (Kerr and Shakespeare, 2002). Sterilisation laws were adopted in parts of Canada, the United States (Kevles, 1985) and all the Nordic countries (Broberg and Roll-Hansen, 1996), as well as in Germany. Under the Nazis, disabled people were persecuted with ruthless efficiency (Gallagher, 1995). Sterilisation was carried out on 5 per cent of the population, and on the outbreak of war a ferocious euthanasia programme lead to the death of 200,000 to 275,000 people, the majority with mental illness or learning difficulties (Burleigh, 1994). Medical professionals were at the forefront of Nazi eugenic and euthanasia programmes (Lifton, 1986).

However, making direct analogies between Nazi programmes and contemporary policy and practice (Disability Awareness in Action, 1997: 1) makes for highly effective rhetoric but dubious argument, as historian Michael Burleigh suggests (1998: 145). The Nazi comparison occurs frequently in the writings of disabled commentators. While there are many problematic aspects to the extension of antenatal screening, it is unhelpful and insulting to see most clinicians as fascists or megalomaniacs. Modern democracies do not have sterilisation laws equivalent to those which all Nordic countries and many US states adopted and implemented between 1911–60 (Broberg and Roll-Hansen, 1996; Kevles, 1985). Ideas about 'racial hygiene' and social Darwinism are no longer acceptable in the mainstream. Contemporary clinical genetics is aimed at preventing and treating genuine illness, rather than 'purifying the population' or eliminating racial and social minorities. When disability rights critics rhetorically resort to the Nazi analogy, it becomes easier for scientists, ethicists and policy-makers to ignore the valid element of the disability critique, and even to exclude disabled people from debates as 'irrational' and 'emotive'.

Moreover, the plot discourse imparts an intentionality and coherence to contemporary policy on reproduction which it does not necessarily possess (Shakespeare, 1999a). The conspiratorialism feeds the idea of a plan by the state, abetted by science, to eliminate all disabled people. But genetic advances are incremental, haphazard, contested and complex. Despite the hyperbole of some genetic researchers, the science is limited, incomplete and uncertain. Very few congenital conditions are detectable through mass antenatal screening. Approximately 2 per cent of all births are affected by congenital abnormality, whereas disabled people comprise 10–20 per cent of the population, suggesting that genetic screening could never seriously reduce the incidence of disability. While there are public health policies which will undoubtedly have the indirect consequence of reducing the numbers of babies born with certain impairments (in particular Down syndrome and neural tube defects), the mechanism is more complicated than a negative eugenic programme. There is no government plan to eliminate disabled people.

In particular, consumer demand plays a significant role in the adoption of testing in pregnancy, and the principle of patient autonomy is central to the modern practice of genetics and obstetrics. Rather than coercive eugenics, individual choice is the mechanism by which genetics is implemented (Hampton, 2005). The role of prospective parents has largely been ignored by disability rights critics of genetics. Often it is prospective parents, not clinicians, who are the active agents in choosing to terminate pregnancy.

Therefore when disabled activists argue that 'Disabled people are under threat for their existence in our modern technological societies. Medical science feels able to flex its muscles and power to abolish all life where the unborn foetus may be imperfect or impaired' (Rock 1996: 121), or that 'disabled people as a distinct group are specifically targeted before they are born. Access to prenatal diagnosis has for many years been driven by the goal of getting rid of certain groups of disabled people, for example those with Down's syndrome or spina bifida' (Disability Awareness in Action, 1997: 1), they are producing a narrative which locates control firmly with doctors, not pregnant women; which suggests that screening is motivated by a eugenic urge to eliminate disabled people; and which obscures the way in which women, and their partners, take responsibility for difficult decisions about their pregnancies (Statham and Solomou, 2001). Yet this is grossly to simplify the complexities of the antenatal encounter.

Paul (1992) shows that the debate about the eugenic nature of contemporary genetics is not ultimately resolvable, because the term 'eugenics' has so many meanings. 'Eugenics' literally means 'well born', and could be broadly defined as any attempt to improve the quality of future generations. But at this level of generality, eugenics includes all those areas of welfare policy which are directed towards improving the well-being of children and families. Eugenics could be defined more narrowly as attempts to influence the distribution of particular undesired genes in the population. This is closer to the common understanding of the term. But conceptually and in practice, this also could imply a range of approaches. Historians distinguish between positive eugenics and negative eugenics (Kevles, 1985). The former involves encouraging reproduction of individuals with preferred characteristics. The latter involves discouraging reproduction of individuals with undesirable characteristics. Another key distinction is between a eugenics which relies on voluntary action, influenced by education and advice, and a coercive eugenics, based on legal controls or paternalistic professional practices (Caplan et al., 1999).

Regardless of emphasis and method, each of these approaches imply eugenic intentions: an agent with eugenic goals who acts to further those goals. In contemporary biomedicine, it is rare to find explicitly eugenic values or programmes promoted (although see Rogers, 1999 for an example). However, another approach would define eugenics in terms of outcomes. It may not be necessary for there to be a eugenic agent, or an explicitly eugenic agenda. As a result of particular social policies and individual choices, eugenic outcomes (a reduction in the births affected by particular conditions) may result. This is what Philip Kitcher (1997) calls 'laissez-faire eugenics' and what Simon Hampton (2005) describes as 'family eugenics'. Many contemporary bioethicists have argued that, as long as there is no coercion involved, this form of eugenics is not objectionable (Caplan et al., 1999). For some, eugenics of this voluntary, consumer or laissez-faire type should be positively endorsed as a moral and social practice (Harris, 1992). However, in my own work (Shakespeare, 1998, 2005a) I have tried to highlight the limitations on choice, suggesting that, even in the absence of explicitly eugenic intentions, eugenics may be an 'emergent property' arising out of the thousands of interactions, implicit expectations, subtle influences and restricted choices in which prospective parents find themselves (McLaughlin, 2003; Hampton, 2005).

The complexities of these issues undermine the sloganising which equates genetics with eugenics, or doctors with Nazis. Eugenics has become a powerful slur word to denounce contemporary practices, but it carries no commonly agreed meaning apart from the general implication that anything eugenic must be bad, because of the historic abuses carried out in the name of eugenics (Wikler, 1999). Complacency about the context in which reproductive decisions are made is misguided. But polemic and conspiracy theory are also misplaced (King, 1999). It is offensive both to physicians and to those prospective parents who agonise long and hard about testing and termination to use highly emotive rhetoric to denounce modern antenatal screening and those who hold different moral positions on abortion or disability.

## Is prenatal diagnosis discriminatory?

The second theme of the disability rights critique eschews the rhetoric of eugenics and conspiracy, and focuses on the meanings and implications of individual choices and biomedical practices (Parens and Asch, 2000). For example, it is claimed that prenatal diagnosis discriminates against foetuses with impairments. A pregnancy which would have continued to term if the foetus had been unaffected is aborted because the foetus has, or is believed to have, a condition which would lead to impairment. Or it may be claimed that prenatal diagnosis discriminates against disabled children and adults, because it sends the message that it would have been better if they, too, had not been born. This argument is often called 'the expressivist objection', because it suggests that genetic diagnosis and selective abortion 'expresses' discriminatory or negative views towards disabled people.

One of the strengths of the expressivist objection is that it forces us to attend to the language of prenatal diagnosis, and the wider messages which it conveys. There are many examples of highly prejudicial language being used about disabled people in the literature on genetics and screening, for example 'culprit chromosomes' and 'random tragedies' (Shakespeare, 1999a). The second important dimension of the expressivist objection is that it captures the extent to which impairment is part of the identity of many disabled people, particularly those with congenital conditions: whereas non-disabled commentators see impairment as a separate aspect (like having influenza), disabled people argue that it is an important aspect of who they are (Edwards, 2004, 2005). Finally, the expressivist objection also highlights the emotional impact of screening programmes on disabled people, and often on those who love and support them. It can be very difficult to accept that a genetic test or screening technology has been developed which might have prevented one's own birth. A person with a congenital impairment immediately imagines whether their own parents would have taken advantage of the technology. It brings up fears about rejection and not being wanted by one's family or society. It makes one think of a society in which one did not exist. All of these are painful and threatening thoughts, made worse by the very negative language in which these technologies are discussed and promoted: as Steve Edwards suggests, 'the moral wrongness of the practice stems from the harmful effects it has' (Edwards, 2004: 419).

Yet, there is a logical contradiction in this emotional response. Any disabled person has already been born. Prior to being born, the disabled person does not exist in any meaningful sense. During the mother's pregnancy, a cluster of developing cells existed, but not a person with identity, experiences and feelings. The response 'I would not have been born' has an emotional resonance, but cannot be understood in strictly rational terms, because before anyone is born, there is no 'I' not to be born. The more logical response is to think 'this technology might prevent future people like myself being born' or 'this may lead to a world in which there are fewer people with conditions like mine'. This may still be experienced as regrettable and distressing, but has less personal resonance than the idea of non-existence.

Moreover, there are many circumstances in which one could imagine a situation in which one would not have been born, as John Harris (1992) and others argue. For example, I would not have been born if my parents had not met; if they had used contraception; if they had made love a month later; indeed, had they made love a millisecond later, I would not have been born. According to Saul Kripke's zygotic principle, each individual is the unique result of one sperm fertilising one egg (unless they are a monozygotic twin), and any other combination or moment of conception would have resulted in a different person – a brother or sister, but not me (Kripke, 1980).

The expressivist objection seems to apply to any technology which limits possible births. For example, people use contraception or sterilisation to avoid having unwanted or further children: do these techniques therefore express negative valuation of children born to unmarried women, or children born into large families? But the expressivists reply, the point about antenatal diagnosis is that it specifies a class of people who are to be avoided. It is the characteristics of the potential child which are diagnosed and which the parents endeavour to avoid. It is the message which screening sends about disability which is so problematic. We need then to turn to the question of whether seeking to prevent disability necessarily expresses a negative valuation of existing disabled people.

## Is it always wrong to prevent impairment?

Contrary to the expressivist objection, I do not believe that attempts to prevent impairment necessarily send negative messages about disabled people. It is not inconsistent to support the rights of existing disabled people, while seeking to prevent more people becoming impaired. For example, any public health programme attempts to minimise the number of people who are disabled. Inoculation of babies or mine clearance schemes are all intended to stop people becoming impaired, but do not therefore imply that people with polio or missing limbs are second class citizens. Of course, there are ways of promoting these morally positive endeavours which do rebound negatively on perceptions of disability. For example, in the late 1990s there was a British anti-drink driving campaigning which used footage of a severely brain damaged man. The hard-hitting message of the advertisement was that viewers risked ending up as a pathetic vegetable if they drove a vehicle under the influence of alcohol. An important piece of health information was conveyed in a way which expressed very negative attitudes towards people with brain injury.

But, in general, most people would accept that because impairment is not a neutral state, but a condition which is generally unwelcome and best avoided, attempts to reduce the numbers of disabled children being born are acceptable, if they are promoted in ways which do not threaten existing disabled children and adults. For example, cerebral palsy is associated with premature births and complications during delivery which cause anoxia, and hence brain damage. Obstetric and neonatal specialists attempt to reduce the incidence of cerebral palsy through improving care of mothers and babies. This does not express a negative valuation of people with cerebral palsy, or have implications for their rights or potentiality. Another example is the policy of promoting folic acid as a dietary supplement. Folate is proven to reduce the incidence of spina bifida during early foetal development. If it was added to flour, as happens in USA, the numbers of pregnancies affected by spina bifida and other malformations would reduce dramatically. This would seem to be straightforwardly a good outcome.

It may be that disability activists who experience spina bifida or cerebral palsy object to these policies. At the Oslo Congress of Rehabilitation International, I met a Ugandan woman who told me that disability activists in her country had criticised polio immunisation programmes, on the grounds that these expressed negative attitudes to disability. Such reactions seem misguided. Many people with polio, cerebral palsy and spina bifida are indeed happy, well-adjusted and successful. All people with these conditions are deserving of rights and respect. But this does not have implications for measures to prevent future people experiencing conditions which can be associated with discomfort and restriction. Impairment prevention does not imply negative valuation of people who already have an impairment, and the two policies – impairment prevention and disability rights – are not incompatible.

However, there is an important distinction which needs to be made. In philosophical terms, these examples are 'same number cases' (Parfit, 1984). Often bioethicists talk in hypothetical terms about a situation in which someone could take a pill, which would prevent or cause impairment in their future child, or perhaps avoid impairment by waiting a month to conceive. In these cases, it is commonly argued that the prospective parent has a moral duty to take the course of action which would result in the healthy, unaffected child. Interventions such as folate, or obstetric and neonatatal care do not prevent the birth of a particular foetus, but instead prevent that foetus being born with impairment. As with inoculation, these practices are about preventing impairment in future people, not preventing potential people who are impaired. As Ruth Bailey observes, to think of prenatal diagnosis in exactly the same terms as these other forms of impairment prevention is wrong:

> This obscures the fundamental difference between prenatal testing and any other way of preventing illness, namely that the 'treatment' which follows prenatal testing – abortion – 'cures' the condition by eliminating the foetus rather than by stopping the condition occurring in the first place.
>
> (Bailey, 1996: 149)

In other words, the force of the expressivist objection does not seem directed against reduction of impairment per se, but against reduction of impairment using abortion as the method. It is this which might send the message that 'it is better to be dead than disabled' and thus expresses a negative valuation of, or misrecognition or disrespect towards, the lives of disabled people. Therefore, we need to examine arguments about the acceptability of termination of pregnancy.

## Is it wrong to terminate pregnancy when the foetus is impaired?

The morality of abortion is complex and contested, and full discussion is beyond the scope of this chapter (see Warren, 1993, for fuller discussion of different positions on abortion). However, I want briefly to explain why I cannot accept the two most extreme responses to the problem, namely the position which argues life starts at conception – and so all abortion is wrong – and the position which says abortion is permissible until birth (on the ground's of a woman's autonomy, or that a baby is not a person).

Some people, including some motivated by disability rights arguments, are opposed to abortion in all circumstances. They do not distinguish between cases where the foetus is disabled, and cases where the foetus is unaffected. They believe that abortion is wrong in all circumstances, because the foetus is a living human being, which is entitled to the rights and respect due to other human beings. Just as it is wrong to kill a baby, child or adult human being, so it is wrong to kill an embryo or foetus as it develops in the womb. Abortion, or embryo research, from this perspective, is murder.

The polar opposite view to the anti-abortionist position is held by those feminists and others who stress a woman's right to choose what happens to her body (Sharp and Earle, 2002). The foetus is part of the woman, and therefore the woman is the only person who has the right to decide what happens to the pregnancy. Either the foetus has no rights, because it is not a person, or the rights of the foetus are trumped by the rights of the woman in whose womb the foetus is developing. The maximalist feminist position suggests that a woman has the right to abortion on demand at any stage up until birth, for any reason.

However, many disability rights commentators take a third position, because while they support the feminist principle of reproductive autonomy, they are anxious about selective termination of impaired foetuses (Asch, 2000; Saxton, 2000). They argue that abortion is allowable if a woman does not want to be pregnant. However, it is not allowable if a woman does not want to be pregnant with this particular foetus. In other words, abortion rights should extend to the choice of becoming a mother or not at a particular time and with a particular partner, but not to any choices which depend on the characteristics of the foetus. The reason often given for this conditional support of abortion rights is that selective termination of impaired foetuses expresses negative valuation of disabled people and/or discriminates against impaired foetuses. A common analogy (for example, Asch and Geller, 1996) is that it is not ethically different to select against girl foetuses than to select against foetuses with genetic disorders. Many people have the intuition that selective termination of female foetuses is wrong, usually because it sends negative messages about the value of women. Opponents of selective termination of impaired foetuses use the same argument about the value of disabled people.

The problem for blanket anti-abortionists, as Ronald Dworkin (1984) has pointed out, is that few of them are totally consistent. For example, many anti-abortionists would permit abortion in cases where the pregnancy has arisen as a consequence of rape. Others would permit abortion in cases where the life of the mother is in danger. Equally, blanket anti-abortionists often do not oppose the taking of life in other circumstances, for example in war or capital punishment. Dworkin concludes that anti-abortionists, although they say they are motivated by a belief that abortion is murder, must be mistaken. If abortion is murder, it remains murder even if the cause of the pregnancy was rape. After all, the foetus is not to blame for the circumstances of its conception. The mother may be very distressed, but it would be possible for her to have the child and give it up for adoption, which would be preferable to murder.

The problem for maximal feminists is that the idea of women having property rights in their bodies and hence the right to decide about their pregnancies ignores the fact that pregnancies affect third parties, not just women. After a certain point in pregnancy – certainly by the third trimester – the interests of the developing baby have to be balanced with those of the pregnant woman. Particularly in the later stage of pregnancy, it seems objectionable that a baby who may be able to survive independently outside the womb has no rights, and the mother is entitled to have it killed. The extreme feminist position has the merit of consistency, but leads to repugnant conclusions.

The problem for the disability rights selective objection to abortion is that it is inconsistent. It seems intuitively true that if it is permissible to terminate pregnancy at all, it is permissible to terminate in the case of disability. It does not make sense to me that it is acceptable to have an abortion for social reasons – for example, the timing of the pregnancy is inconvenient, or the woman does not want a baby with this particular man, or the prospective parents do not want another addition to their family – but not for the morally significant reason that the foetus is affected by an impairment. Moreover, it is only possible to speak of discrimination against impaired foetuses if they are humans entitled to full moral rights, and if this is the case, all abortion is wrong, not just abortion of impaired foetuses (Warren, 1997).

Two examples further erode the disability rights movement's opposition to selecting on the basis of fetal characteristics. First, there are many cases of profound impairment, where the prospective life is very seriously affected, where disability rights critics often waive their objection: for example, metabolic disorders such as Tay-Sachs disease, where babies usually die by by the age of five or Lesch-Nyhan syndrome, where the child may grow to young adulthood, but in a state of very severe physical and mental distress. If these are situations in which diagnosis can be taken into account, the general principle that it is wrong to choose on the basis of foetal characteristics is undermined. Second, a situation could be imagined when a young single woman becomes pregnant and is considering whether to have an abortion. For a woman of 16 or 17, the characteristics of the foetus could be very relevant to her decision. She might think that she could possibly cope with a child, knowing that support will be available, that childcare will be available, and that she has a chance of continuing her education and achieving a good quality of life for herself and her baby. Contrast this with her prospects if she has a baby with a serious impairment. There may not be enough support, there may not be appropriate childcare, and it may be almost impossible for her to achieve her aspirations. The future for both her and the child might be very bleak. To this young woman, the question of the characteristics of the foetus are not separable from, or irrelevant to, the question of whether she continues the pregnancy.

Unlike the blanket anti-abortionists, and many of the maximalist feminists, I hold the gradualist position (Gillon, 2001). This suggests that the developing foetus should be regarded as having increasing moral status as pregnancy progresses. The early embryo has potential, but it is not a full human being with all the status and protection which that implies (the analogy of the acorn versus the oak is sometimes used). The third trimester baby may still be in the womb, but has a good chance of viability, and is in most morally significant respects a person with human rights. Gradualism is a tenuous answer to the abortion question, because it is difficult to state exactly when the transition to moral status occurs. Significance is often attached to biological milestones – such as the capacity for sentience or viability outside the womb, both of which occur at the earliest between 20–24 weeks.

Beyond these metaphysical and legal questions, it is important to add that abortion is neither a tragedy (as many anti-abortionists claim) nor an insignificant clinical procedure (as some pro-choice activists claim). All termination or loss of pregnancy, at any stage, may be sad and regrettable, because it involves the extinction of a growing human life, full of potential and promise. In particular, psychological evidence suggests that the termination of a wanted pregnancy after diagnosis of foetal abnormality at 18–20 weeks is associated with guilt and distress on the part of the parents who have to make that difficult choice, especially the prospective mother. The pain may continue for many years, perhaps even a lifetime (White-van Mourik, 1994).

While the gradualist position can be interpreted as supporting general access to first trimester termination, with second trimester termination in circumstances of foetal anomaly, third trimester termination is morally very contentious. It is at this point that a disability rights claim of unfair discrimination does have purchase. Current UK law on abortion states that it is prohibited after the 24th week of pregnancy, except in cases where there is a substantial risk that the child would be born 'seriously handicapped' (Shakespeare, 1998; Sheldon and Wilkinson, 2001). In other words, third trimester foetuses are protected in law, unless they are at risk of impairment, in which case they are not protected until birth (and not always then). A simple charge of discrimination (Shakespeare, 1998) fails, because here a distinction is being made on morally relevant grounds: a foetus with serious impairment is different from a healthy foetus, and to some this relevant difference is a sufficient reason for overturning usual protections. Others resolve the inconsistency (or discrimination) by arguing in favour of permitting late termination for any pregnancy, not just pregnancies affected by impairment (Savulescu, 2001). I find this objectionable, because to me a third trimester foetus has moral status.

In practice, late abortion necessitates foeticide. After 24 weeks, a baby is viable outside the womb, given medical care. At this point, if birth is induced, the baby would be born alive, and hence doctors would be compelled to attempt to keep it alive (although some utilitarians argue this is unnecessary). The differences between most impaired foetuses and non-impaired foetuses do not seem sufficient to justify such killing of an otherwise viable baby. The legal loophole permitting late abortions was intended to cover the very small number of cases where the foetus was non-viable (likely to die in pregnancy or soon after birth), but seems to have been exploited in other cases where the impairment was not incompatible with life (notoriously, in one instance a case of cleft lip and palate; see Allison, 2003). For these reasons, it seems to me urgently important to tighten UK law so that late termination is only permissable where the life of the mother is in danger, or when it is inevitable that the foetus will die before birth or in the neonatal period.

While first and second trimester prenatal diagnosis and selective abortion is regrettable and distressing for prospective parents, it is hard to claim that it is morally wrong or should be further prohibited. We live in an age where scientific knowledge can provide information about the characteristics of the developing baby. Where there is evidence of a serious condition which may cause considerable suffering or restriction to the future child, and difficulties and restrictions for other family members, a utilitarian would argue that it is not wrong to enable pregnant women and their partners to exercise their right to access abortion: by doing so, they make their own lives easier, and reduce the amount of suffering in the world (Glover, 1977; Harris, 1992).

By contrast, virtue ethicists discuss selection abortion in terms of the moral character of the parents, and which decisions are compatible with good parenting (Macintyre, 1999; Vehmas, 2002). Rather than discussing parental duties or foetal rights, virtue ethics emphasises parental responsibility, and the unconditional love of a parent for his child. For example, Macintyre argues that the virtuous parent is orientated towards the child's needs, not their own needs, whatever those needs may turn out to be. 'Good parental care is defined in part by reference to the possibility of the affliction of their children by serious disability' (Macintyre, 1999: 91). For him, parents of disabled children are the paradigms of good parenthood, 'who provide the model for and the key to the work of all parents' (1999: 91). To me, the virtue ethics position has more purchase after the birth of a disabled child than in pregnancy when serious impairment is predicted. Macintyre is perhaps over-idealistic about the virtues of good parenting. Because I cannot accept that abortion prior to 20 weeks is morally wrong, it seems to me that abortion on the grounds of serious impairment must also be justifiable.

Abortion is a moral harm, because it involves killing and the deprivation of a future of value to the foetus (Savulescu, 2002). This harm has to be compared with the moral harm of avoidable impairment (Glover, 1977). The equation will play out differently for different people, depending on the resources they have available to them, the seriousness of the impairment, their beliefs about their own capabilities, and their view of what makes a good life. These are difficult positions, which are the private responsibility and concern of individual women and men, and should be discussed with humility and caution by philosophers, activists and others who do not have to live with the consequences.

*[handwritten note in left margin: I can agree w this.]*

## Will selective termination of impaired foetuses harm existing disabled people?

The expressivist argument could be interpreted in non-consequentialist and consequentialist ways (Michael Parker, personal communication): the former suggests that termination reflects or expresses a discriminatory attitude, and that this would be wrong even if no disabled person was negatively affected. In other words, some motivations for selective termination are wrong, even if selective termination is not always wrong. However, the latter and more powerful version of expressivism grounds the wrongness of selective termination in the harms that result as a consequence: the implications are that other people will have to live with the consequences of decisions to terminate pregnancies affected by impairment, not just the parents. It is claimed that there will be negative consequences for disabled people, if policies and practices which allow people to terminate pregnancy to avoid having disabled children are permitted.

Clearly, many disabled people and their supporters feel offended by prenatal diagnosis. But this does not mean that prenatal diagnosis is wrong: as Steve Edwards claims, 'One is obliged to take into account consequences of one's actions which might harm others, but it does not follow that those harms count for more than the suppression of one's free choice' (Edwards, 2004: 419). While there is evidence that some disabled people feel offended and discriminated against by prenatal diagnosis, there is no strong empirical evidence that material harms to disabled people result from selective abortion. For example, the increase in prenatal diagnosis and selective abortion does not seem to have resulted in a worsening of attitudes towards disabled people, or a reduction in standards of care, or quality of life. On the contrary, the irony is that the increasing availability of genetic knowledge has coincided with the increasing acceptance of disability rights and slowly improving provision for disabled people.

Disability rights activists assume that abortion on the basis of impairment suggests that it would be better to be dead than disabled. However, as Anne Maclean and many others have argued, there is a distinction to be made between abortion suggesting that disabled people's lives are not worth living, and a case where an individual person cannot cope with a disabled child (Maclean, 1993). For example, parents may feel that having a disabled child will damage their partnership, or impact negatively on their other children. They may fear economic hardship, particularly if one parent has to give up working to care for the disabled child. They may be prepared to sacrifice freedoms in order to parent children for the first twenty years of the children's lives, but not to continue in a parental role towards an adult disabled child who remains dependent. There are many extra-ordinary stories of the degree of selflessness and commitment which Macintyre calls for, and such people should certainly be welcomed and applauded. But not all prospective parents will be prepared to make the sacrifices and endure the difficulties that disabled families sometimes face, and it is their right to forgo this future, which does not imply that they do not like, respect and accept disabled people.

It might even be argued that selective abortion can benefit existing disabled people. For example, some couples both carry a recessive genetic condition, which causes a risk of serious impairment – such as cystic fibrosis – in their children. They may only discover their risk as a result of having an affected child. Much as they love that child, they may decide that they cannot cope with another disabled child, and use prenatal diagnosis to avoid that possibility. The benefit to the existing child is that the parents can concentrate their attention and care on him, and do not have to try and support two children with high support needs. This example also shows that it is compatible to love and respect an existing disabled person, while taking steps to ensure that the impairment does not recur.

This claim should not be confused with an implicit reason that is sometimes given for selective termination. Advocates of screening – or indeed prospective parents – may believe it is in the interests of the potential disabled child not to be born, because life with impairment causes suffering or restriction (Glover, 1977). The question of whether a foetus has interests is complex and contested (Sheldon and Wilkinson, 2001: 89). However, it seems plausible that it is always in the interests of a potential person to be born, unless the life they would lead is worse than not existing at all (Harris, 2000). Very few forms of impairment involve so much suffering that non-existence would be preferable. In other words, prenatal diagnosis can be justified in terms of the effect on parents and other siblings, but cannot be justified in terms of the benefits to the life which is prevented from coming into existence as a result, except in the most severe cases of impairment. A child is not harmed by being born, which is why 'wrongful birth' litigation should not be permissible (Spriggs and Savulescu, 2002).

In contrast, opponents of screening argue that the person who is harmed by selective termination is the foetus with impairment. But if this is the basis on which disability rights advocates oppose selective termination, then the position has broader implications. For example, if they argue that impaired foetuses are persons, and thus that selective termination is discrimination towards, or harm to, disabled people, then their position is not just opposed to selective termination, but to all termination. If an impaired foetus is a person who is entitled to protection, then any and each foetus is a person entitled to protection, and thus all abortion has to be murder (Gillon, 2001: ii8).

Above, I have tried to demonstrate that preventing impairment is not wrong in principle. I have argued that the expressivist objection is not a strong reason for prohibiting screening. It is not incompatible to seek to prevent impaired children coming into the world, and also to support the rights of existing disabled people (Buchanan, 1996). I have further suggested that the expressivist objection has the implication that abortion in general is wrong. It appears to me inconsistent and illogical to support abortion rights in all circumstances except where the foetus is likely to grow into a disabled person. Abortion, on any grounds, is morally serious, but during the first and second trimester of pregnancy I believe that the choice should be a legal right, which is left to the individual conscience to decide.

## Is there a duty to diagnose and terminate pregnancies affected by impairment?

Some commentators have argued that prenatal diagnosis is not just permissible, but also obligatory. Others have suggested that prospective parents have a duty not just to test during pregnancy, but also to terminate a pregnancy if the foetus is found to be affected by impairment. For example, the IVF pioneer Professor Robert Edwards has stated, 'In the future, it will be a sin to have a disabled child' (Rogers, 1999). It should be noted that pronouncements of this kind, though rare, are of exactly the same form as the pre-1945 eugenics which society more generally repudiates.

The range of spiritual and ethical views as to the acceptability of abortion suggests to me that neither society nor the state can prescribe the course of action an individual should take during pregnancy. The principle of reproductive autonomy suggests that prenatal diagnosis and termination should be available, within certain agreed moral limits, for those who wish freely to avail themselves of it. Society's role consists in providing information, counselling, support and high quality professional services to help safely deliver the chosen outcomes.

What could be the basis of any duty to test or terminate pregnancy? It has already been established that a disabled child is not harmed by being brought into existence, where the only other alternative was not to exist at all, unless the impairment is so severe that it is worse than death. Prospective mothers do have a duty to take all reasonable steps (folate supplement, forgoing excess alcohol and drugs) to ensure that they do not damage a foetus during pregnancy (a future person), but this cannot extend to preventing the birth of an impaired child (a potential person). However, John Harris (1992) and others argue that there are wrongs which are not harms to individuals: creating disabled children, on this account, is wrong because it increases suffering or decreases utility.

Thus, it could be argued that the prospective parents have a duty to society or to the state not to have a disabled child. It is in the interests of society to have productive and healthy citizens, and therefore testing and termination of poten-tially impaired or unhealthy babies is required. This is classic eugenics, and contrary to justice, human rights, and the reproductive rights of parents. A more important objection draws on evidence that many disabled children grow into productive adults with good quality of life (and, indeed, many non-disabled children grow up into unhappy adults with poor quality of life). The idea of disability as automatically equivalent to burden and suffering cannot be sustained empirically (Albrecht and Devlieger, 1999; Brouwer *et al.*, 2005). Although it could be conceded that there will be a small proportion of disabled people who may never be productive, and who may need care throughout their lives, how much of a problem is this in a prosperous western society? Subordinating personal morality and individual human rights to collective interests can only be justified in extreme cases of emergency, which do not pertain in the prenatal diagnosis scenario. The social and economic burden of dependent disabled people in advanced economies is small, compared to expenditure on other items – for example, military spending.

Moreover, if parents have a duty to avoid disability or poor quality of life in their offspring, there are contentious implications. For example, there are other social groups whose offspring may be perceived to be a burden in society: for example, socially excluded communities in the inner cities. But to suggest that such social groups might have a duty not to have children would be regarded as outrageous and offensive by most people. The relevant point about socially excluded people – or about minority ethnic communities who experience racism and consequently a poor quality of life – is that the disadvantage is a consequence of social arrangements. Rather than preventing the birth of people who experience oppression, every energy should be devoted towards removing the source of the social exclusion. Exactly the same argument is made by disability rights advocates. A more supportive and inclusive environment will enable more people with impairment to be independent and productive. Therefore, rather than individual parents having a duty to avoid the birth of disabled children, should it not be society which has a duty to welcome and include disabled children and adults, so that the social problem of disability can be mitigated or eliminated?

In conclusion, there can be no duty to diagnose or prevent impairment in pregnancy. It would be untrue to claim that people with impairments suffer while people without impairments do not suffer or become burdens. All lives involve suffering and dependency, and the only way to avoid suffering is to forgo reproduction entirely. All decisions about screening and termination are difficult, and can only be made by those people who have to live with the consequences – either the distress of abortion, or the potential stress of supporting a disabled child, or an additional child. Society should support people to make good decisions, and support them with the consequences of their decisions. In particular, justice demands that the state should devote more resources to supporting families with disabled children, and to promoting the well-being of disabled adults, rather than acting as if prenatal diagnosis or other biomedical interventions will solve the problem of disability. As Abby Lippman argues,

> Social conditions are as enabling or disabling as biological conditions. Why are biological variations that create differences between individuals seen as

preventable or avoidable while social conditions that create similar distinctions are likely to be seen as intractable givens?

(Lippman, 1994: 160)

## Is prenatal diagnosis a real choice?

In this chapter, I have articulated a liberal position on prenatal diagnosis, which runs counter to the oppositional rhetoric of some disability rights campaigners. However, this does not mean being naive about choice, or about the context in which prospective parents make their choices. I do not believe that there is a coherent drive to eliminate disability from the population. But there are undoubtedly problems with how screening is offered and choices are communicated (Shakespeare, 1998; Hampton, 2005). In this final section, I will explore the contexts in which pregnant women and their partners make their decisions, in order to demonstrate that choices may not be as free as clinical rhetoric suggests. These comprise the 'near patient context' and the 'broader cultural context'.

By the former, I refer to how women and men experience pregnancy services and the offer of screening (Rapp, 1997). There are three areas in which choice may be undermined. The first is information. A good decision depends on relevant and high quality information, which is communicated clearly and understood by the patient. Over many years, social and psychological research has cast doubt on the availability of adequate information in screening (Shakespeare, 1998; McLaughlin, 2003). Work by the National Screening Committee is beginning to standardise the offer of screening across the country, so that all pregnant women are given access to good quality technology, regardless of postcode. Yet this work has not yet been matched by good quality information. In particular, screening information cannot simply be about the experience of having a test, the technical details of the test, and the reliability of the test. The most important question is what the test is for: in other words, information about the conditions which the screening programme is intended to enable women to avoid, if they so choose.

Good quality, balanced information about Down syndrome, spina bifida and other conditions detectable through ultrasound scan, chorion villus sample or amniocentesis is rarely available (Williams *et al.*, 2005). Failure to offer this information carries the implication that it is obvious that someone would want to avoid these conditions, the only question being whether the test is effective in providing the diagnosis. Providing negative information, or information limited to a shallow clinical description of the features of the impairment, carries the implication that the condition is a medical problem which is best avoided (Alderson, 2001). Only if full information about the lives of people who have the condition and their families is provided can prospective parents make an informed decision as to whether they wish to avoid this possibility in their own family. One of the few sources of such antenatal screening information, at the time of writing, is the ANSWER website developed by myself and my team, the pilot version of which provides information about Down syndrome, spina bifida, Turner's syndrome,

Klinefelter's syndrome and cystic fibrosis, based on interviews and photographs of a range of people affected by each condition (www.antenataltesting.info).

The second 'near patient' context which may undermine choice is the attitude and behaviour of medical professionals. If midwives, obstetricians and others working in maternity services imply that women have a duty to have tests or terminations, or if they are unsupportive to women who decline the screening offer, or if they are prejudiced about disability then, clearly, choice is undermined. There is evidence that professionals are frequently directive in this way, particularly from international surveys, but also sometimes in research in the UK (Wertz, 1998; Mao, 1998; Shakespeare, 1998). The majority of professionals may be non-directive and pro-choice, but individuals remain who make it clear to pregnant women that they believe screening to be a great benefit which no sensible person could refuse.

The third element of the 'near patient context' is the routinisation of maternity and screening services. While obstetrics has successfully minimised maternal and infant mortality, this has been at the cost of the autonomy of pregnant women. Screening becomes a conveyor belt, and choice is consequently undermined (Press and Browner, 1997). Another example is obstetric ultrasound (Williams *et al.*, 2005). The purpose of costly scans during pregnancy is not just to reassure women, enable parents to bond with their babies, or provide pretty pictures for relatives. It is also to detect foetal anomalies, so that termination of pregnancy may be offered. Nothing necessarily wrong with that, except that couples may not be clearly informed that they are having a diagnostic test which in a tiny proportion of cases may lead to a heart-rending choice about ending a wanted pregnancy.

By 'broader cultural context', I refer to cultural and social knowledge and attitudes to disability and parenthood. Prospective parents may be largely ignorant about disability. They may not know any disabled people. They may not be aware of the transformations in opportunities and rights which disabled people have experienced. They may still think that disability is 'a fate worse than death', and they may fear their own loss of health and ability. They may not be able to imagine parenting a disabled child, and may fear that the life of a disabled child may be marked by suffering and restriction. These fears may be reinforced by negative cultural stereotypes, and by messages about the benefits of genetic research and prenatal screening. A disabled person who cannot achieve qualifications, or look normal, or have a good career, or live independently may be regarded very negatively in contemporary society. All of these psychological and cultural factors may operate to undermine the possibility of a prospective parent choosing freely (Hampton, 2005). Moroever, as more and more people choose to test and terminate, it will become harder for others to resist and reject selection (Beck-Gernsheim, 1990). I do not suggest that individuals are brainwashed or coerced. However, they may often be fearful and ignorant and sometimes prejudiced. For these reasons, achieving true choice in screening depends on a more extensive debate about the rights and potential of disabled people, and about the duty of society to accept and support those who need help and cannot achieve full independence.

## Conclusion

In this chapter, I have attempted to clarify complex arguments about a very emotive and painful issue in contemporary society. Ironically, both those who oppose and those who advocate prenatal diagnosis can make the mistake of exaggerating the potential of screening to detect and eliminate disabled children. Genetic intervention is not the solution to the disability problem, nor is it a significant threat to disabled people. Only about 10–20 per cent of disabled people have congenital conditions, most of which would not be detected through screening. Technological and economic constraints mean that very few potential conditions are diagnosable. While pre-implantation genetic diagnosis (PGD or embryo selection, sometimes labelled 'designer baby technology') enables detection of more conditions, only a handful of couples each year have PGD in the UK because it is costly, complex and unreliable. PGD technology is closely regulated by the Human Fertilisation and Embryology Authority. The only people who are likely to have access to the service are those with a history of severe genetic disease – for example, recessive conditions such as cystic fibrosis and muscular dystrophy – or who have chromosomal anomalies which make it unlikely that they carry a pregnancy to term. Therefore, while interesting dilemmas are raised (Zeiler, 2005), in terms of disability rights this option seems less problematic than existing prenatal diagnosis (contra King, 1999). For this reason, the analysis in this chapter has concentrated on ubiquitious screening in pregnancy, where the problems of informed consent and emergent eugenics may potentially arise.

I conclude that prenatal diagnosis is not straightforwardly eugenic or discriminatory. While the *practice* of prenatal diagnosis certainly requires reform in the UK, and probably even more so in certain other jurisdictions, the *principle* should not be objectionable or contrary to disability rights. Central to the issue of prenatal diagnosis is the difficult question of abortion. Avoiding impairment is not necessarily problematic, but ending developing life in the womb usually is. As a gradualist, I argue that termination is permissible in the early stage of pregnancy, and believe that diagnosis of significant impairment is one of the grounds which justifies the moral seriousness of abortion. Testing should be limited to serious conditions which undermine quality of life for individuals and families (Henn, 2000). However, the privacy of those faced with these difficult decisions should be respected, and their autonomy supported. Everyone has an interest in helping prospective parents make better decisions, which they are less likely to regret at a future date. We should be on hand to offer counselling, good quality information, and support, but we should not venture to dictate where the duties of prospective parents may lie. Nor should we interpret a decision to have a test or a termination as expressing disrespect or discrimination towards disabled people. Choices in pregnancy are painful and may be experienced as burdensome, but they are not incompatible with disability rights.

# Chapter 7

# Just around the corner
## The quest for cure

While issues at the beginning of life and end of life are most controversial in the bioethics of disability, there is another relevant class of questions which concerns the acceptability or otherwise of attempts to prevent or cure impairment. The imagery of miracle cures is central to cultural representations of disability and medical research, and recent decades have seen an expansion of such coverage with the Human Genome Project, gene therapy and stem cell research. Disability activists and disability studies writers have challenged the obsession with cure, arguing that:

1   Disability is about social barriers and social oppression, not impairment.
2   The priority is structural change, not altering individuals to conform to social norms.
3   Cure discourse individualises and pathologises impairment, which should be understood in terms of difference, not deficit.

In this chapter I interrogate the debate around cure, challenging both the mainstream approach to medical research, and the disability rights response to it. After outlining some mainstream disability studies response to medical research, I explore the principle of cure, and show how the diversity of impairment experiences makes it dangerous to generalise about disabled people's views. Next, I look at some of the practical issues which make the rhetoric and practice of cure problematic, focusing on stem cell research and the role of Christopher Reeve. Then I discuss some difficult cases, before concluding by placing the cure debate within the broader context of bioethics and disability rights.

Three arguments from Part I of the book are relevant to this chapter. First, I argued that a progressive response to disability needs to devote attention to the problem of impairment, which plays an important part in the lives of many disabled people. Second, I argued that a multi-level approach was needed to tackle the disability problem, one which recognised that medical interventions to treat or minimise impairment were valuable, alongside (and not as replacements for) interventions at the social and structural levels. Third, I criticised the reliance on an ethnic conception of disability identity. This is relevant here because some disability rights activists challenge attempts to prevent or cure impairment because they see it as a threat to their own existance, or as expressing the view that their lives are not valid.

## The disability movement on cure

Disability rights organisations and activists sceptical about or opposed to gene therapy or stem cell research have sometimes found themselves in uneasy alliance with anti-abortion voices concerned about embryo research. However, most disability activists are not anti-abortion, and their concern arises from the broader opposition to cure (Leipoldt, 2005; Beresford and Wilson, 2002). This scepticism is usually not couched in explicitly anti-research terms. For example, the official statement of the British Council of Disabled People argues that social model approaches are not incompatible with medical research:

> only on the crudest reading of the social model could it be argued that this model is about rejecting medical treatment or research. The medical model itself is not about medical intervention, but rather the medicalisation of disabled people. This is what we reject . . . We are also not making a case against medical research, but rather one for a more equitable distribution of effort and resources in order that a real difference can be made now in the lives of disabled people (British Council of Disabled People n.d.).

Goggin and Newell (2004: 51) have discussed what they call the 'mythical structure' of the stem cell debate, in the Australian context. They argue that stem cell therapy is seen as deliverance from catastrophe. The underlying assumptions of this mythic structure are:

- disability individualised, not created by society;
- people with disabilities to be acted upon;
- technology as both value neutral and beneficent;
- magnification of voices supportive of the technology;
- heroic delivery of us from disability as moral trump card;
- technology deals with disability: political issues not needed.

Neither of these accounts seems to be based on an intrinsic objection to stem cell research, unlike the faith-based opponents. Instead, there is a resentment about the prioritisation of medical approaches to the disability problem, and what is seen as a neglect of contextual approaches to the disability problem. These critiques highlight the unbalanced coverage of disability, claiming that media fascination with unproven research leads to a neglect of political issues. Medical therapies are definitely unproven, perhaps impossible, and in any case inappropriate given the everyday problems of disabled people. Neither account acknowledges that a successful medical therapy would be a good outcome: both bracket the issue of potential clinical benefit, either by saying that cure is impossible, or by ignoring the possibility in favour of more political questions.

Underlying these critiques is the prevailing disability rights unwillingness to engage with the question of impairment. Whereas the narrative of cure sees disabled people as people with impairments, the social model approach sees disabled people as victims of social oppression and exclusion. To focus on curing impairment is to challenge the whole basis of the social model story about disability, and therefore it becomes unacceptable (Oliver, 1989). It often appears that what is at stake in these bitterly fought arguments about medical cures are competing identity narratives.

Many disability rights accounts of medical research focus on hype, and claim to be opposed not to cure itself, but to irresponsible promises and raised expectations. For example, the newsletter *Disability Awareness in Action* special report on biotechnology says:

> Few of us would be opposed to research that holds the promise of finding cures for humankind's killer diseases – although we should be aware of the difficulty in separating what can be achieved from what scientists hope will be achieved.
> (Disability Awareness in Action, n.d.)

Michael Oliver's inaugural professorial lecture, 'What's so wonderful about walking?' (republished in *Understanding Disability*, 1996) gives a more sustained analysis and critique of the hyping of medical research. At the outset of his lecture, Oliver quotes from his first published sociological paper, 'the aim of research should not be to make the legless normal, whatever that might mean, but to create a social environment where to be legless is irrelevant' (Oliver, 1978, quoted in Oliver, 1996: 137). He goes on to describe medical research charities as forms of millenarian movement, which he defines as 'a collective this-worldly movement promising total social change by miraculous means' (Oliver, 1996: 100) He is deeply sceptical about the track record of medical research:

> The problem is of course, that throughout the history of humankind, the number of cures that have been found to these 'chronic and crippling diseases' could be counted on the fingers of one hand and still leave some over to eat your dinner with.
> (Oliver, 1996: 101)

In particular, he criticises the International Spinal Research Trust, which in 1986 was promising cures for spinal cord injury within five years. In other publications, Oliver (1989) has compared conductive education, a therapy for children with cerebral palsy, to Nazism and child abuse. However, these criticisms prompted a backlash from people directly involved, arguing that some of the Peto interventions can generate significant outcomes for people with these impairments (Beardshaw, 1989; Read, 1998).

It is not clear whether these challenges reflect the attitudes of disabled people in general. The only survey of disability activists, conducted on behalf of RADAR by Agnes Fletcher (1999), found considerable support for genetic research which might result in cures for impairment and illness: 73 per cent of respondents believed it would be great if new genetic treatments could be developed for conditions like cystic fibrosis or muscular dystrophy. It is clear that there are a range of views on the principle of cure, and on specific therapies. While it is important that disabled voices are heard in the debate, it is misleading to assume that disabled people will speak with one voice.

## The principle of cure

One reason for the diversity of views in the disability community is the diversity of impairment experiences among disabled people. The particular experience of impairment will influence an individual's attitudes to disability and to medicine. This is not to claim that two people with the same impairment will have the same views, but instead to make the broad generalisation that the complexity of impairment effects contributes to disagreement among disabled people.

For example, people with congenital impairments which are largely static in nature tend to be well-adjusted to their situation, partly because they have known no other state. Impairment is their normality, and people may be very well adapted to their situation. Other family members may have their condition, due to genetic factors, and they may associate with other people with the same condition. In this context, impairment becomes a part of personal identity, to the point that the individual cannot conceive of themselves without their impairment (Edwards, 2005). Development of a positive sense of self may depend on a positive reading of impairment, which is revalued in a community based on difference. The classic examples of such impairments include restricted growth, blindness and Deafness. However, many people with cerebral palsy and other conditions present from birth may also value their difference as part of their identity.

In this situation, there may be little enthusiasm for cures, and indeed complete cures for these conditions are unlikely. Corrective surgery in childhood may have been experienced very negatively. Cure may be seen as irrelevant or even threatening and politically offensive. While there is often a worsening of health states due to age, the conditions are not associated with premature mortality or major health complications. People may be different – for example, people with Down syndrome – and even restricted in their choices and abilities, but they generally adapt well to their situation, and minimise the role of impairment in their lives.

Compare this with those who have acute degenerative conditions. Some of these conditions may have been present at birth due to genetic inheritance, but often they only become problematic during childhood, or else they are acquired in midlife. The individual may have known normal functioning, or at least better functioning: they may have appeared normal, rather than different and disabled. People subsequently experience health problems and degeneration of physical and sometimes mental state. Impairment may not be seen as part of personal identity: it may be seen as an external threat, or as an illness for which cure is keenly sought. The classic examples of this group of impairments are multiple sclerosis, muscular dystrophy, Friedriech's ataxia and similar rare genetic conditions. HIV/AIDS has many similarities. In these situtions, there may be considerable interest, even a desperation, for cures (see, for example, patient views expressed in the journal Euroataxia at www.euro-ataxia.org).

A third group are those who develop impairments as a result of the ageing process. This may be the largest section of the disabled population, covering conditions such as arthritis and rheumatism, heart disease, strokes and Parkinsonism. Many people with these conditions may see impairment and restriction as a normal part of ageing. They are less likely to identify as disabled or as part of the disability community, retaining their lifelong sense of themselves as normal. Impairment will be regarded as a pathology. They are likely to want rid of their impairment or illness – particularly if it has been of rapid onset – but many will be resigned to their situation and have low expectations of cure.

Finally, there is the group of those who have acquired static impairment in midlife, for example people with spinal cord injury. Like the late-life acquirers, this group have lived normal lives, and sudden impairment may be unfamiliar and devestating. They may be able to separate their identity from impairment for a time, which may make the process of adaptation more difficult. Once rehabilitation is complete, they do not identify as ill, because they have a static state. The main limiting factors may be experienced as social barriers and social attitudes. However, there may be subsequent degeneration as the ageing process sets in (as with post-polio syndrome). People in this group vary in their identity: some deny their difference, seeking normality; others take the radical disability identity route; others feel defined by their impairment, which they continue to see as pathology and hence seek cure. For example, Michael Oliver is a famous case of a tetraplegic claiming that his injury had a positive impact on his life, and that he would not want a cure, while Smith and Sparkes (2004) discuss a group of men with spinal cord injury, the majority of whom were very definitely 'waiting for the cure'.

This brief sketch of four experiences of impairment/disability shows that individuals will differ in the extent to which they normalise impairment, and the extent to which it becomes part of their identity. The complexity of this debate increases further when different types of cure or therapy are considered. Complete elimination of impairment or disease state is very improbable for most disabled people (although medical successes with childhood leukaemia and other illnesses should not be ignored). However, there is a range of interventions which have changed the experience of impairment over the past century. For example, immunisation has limited infectious diseases such as smallpox and polio. Understandings of disease processes have minimised other conditions through prenatal interventions: for example, phenylketoneuria is a genetic condition which leads to severe learning difficulties, but a simple blood test after birth identifies vulnerable infants, who are placed on an exclusion diet and therefore can attain normal functioning. Administering folate before conception and in the early stages of pregnancy similarly reduces the incidence of spina bifida. Against these successes are the scandals of pharmaceuticals which have actually generated impairment, most notoriously Thalidomide, but also other teratogens such as anti-epilepsy drugs.

Another class of interventions enable the affected individual to gain better life expectancy, although they do not cure the impairment. In public health terms, a reduction in mortality is associated with a gain in morbidity. For the individuals concerned, this is obviously a major benefit, and is evidence that the cure rhetoric has some validity. For example, new understandings of diabetes and insulin in the 1920s led to the survival of those who developed type one diabetes. Spinal cord injury was associated with premature mortality, until better management after World War II enabled paralysed people to achieve normal life expectancy. Similarly, heart/lung transplants have increased life expectancy for many people with cystic fibrosis, and the simple technique of nocturnal ventilation has enabled longer survival of young men with Duchenne muscular dystrophy (Eagle *et al.*, 2002). The use of combination therapies has converted HIV/AIDS from an acute terminal illness into a chronic condition.

Many of these beneficial interventions enable people with illness or impairment to move from one disease state to another. For example, spinal stabilisation enables some people with spinal cord injury to have a partial rather than total break of spinal nerves. Gene therapy has successfully cured severe combined immune deficiency in some children, although some have subsequently developed leukaemia (Marwick 2003). Current gene therapy research aims to convert Duchenne muscular dystrophy into a less severe variant of the disease. Some interventions for people with sensory deficits cannot cure deafness or blindness, but can achieve gains in sensory function which are experienced as improvements.

Another class of intervention is targeted at improving functioning or quality of life. For example, pacemakers, cochlear implants, hip replacements have all been experienced positively by people who were previously limited by their physical condition. Surgical interventions such as limb-straightening have enabled restricted growth people with bow legs or malformed joints to be more mobile and avoid worsening of their conditions. People with cerebral palsy have taken muscle relaxing drugs which reduce spasm. Prozac and other SSRI drugs have enabled people at risk of depression to function more effectively day-to-day.

Finally, there are those interventions which seem more designed to normalise or provide cosmetic improvements than to tackle an underlying functional problem. For example, cosmetic surgery for people with Down syndrome, limb-lengthening for people with restricted growth, or other aesthetic surgery or orthopedic interventions. Here an individual – or their family members – facing negative social reaction seeks medical help to minimise difference and fit in. From a disability rights perspective, these interventions may be seen as 'blaming the victim'. Rather than solving the disability problem by removing social barriers, the individual is corrected to fit in with the norm. However, often interventions have both social and functional benefits. Sometimes it is unrealistic to expect major social or cultural change, and in the meantime seemingly cosmetic interventions can improve quality of life. Negative social judgements may also be based on the dangerous assumption that psychological problems are not as serious as physical problems.

This sketch of different impairment states, and different aspects of cure and therapy, was not intended to achieve a systematic analysis of the field. However, it is sufficient to show the considerable variety of experiences, reactions and interventions, and to challenge simplistic generalisations or blanket political opposition. People have different reasons for turning to medicine, and will have different reactions to their own impairment. Moroever, some cultures will be more supportive of difference than others.

Nor is medical cure or therapy incompatible with social change and civil rights: rather than seeing these as alternative strategies, it is possible to see them as complementary. For example, De Wolfe, who experiences ME, has called for recognition of the importance of cure, and the expansion of the social model to include illness:

> Most people who feel continuously weak, tired, giddy, in pain, will inevitably construe themselves as potential clients of curative medicine. By contrast with certain impairments discussed by disability activists, illness often does constitute tragedy, both for its victims and for those close to them.
>
> (De Wolfe, 2002: 261)

Yet this is not to deny that social arrangements also make a big difference.

Almost all disabled people, even where they are happy with the way they are, are unwilling to loose further function: while they may not want a cure, they do not want to lose the abilities they have currently, or have their health state worsen. For this reason, it seems to me that it is misguided to oppose cures and therapies in principle: each should be taken on its merits.

## Cures in practice

However, while cure may be theoretically acceptable, there might be problems in practice. For example, cures may be inappropriate responses to the challenge of disability, either because the person is not experiencing their difference negatively, or because barrier removal or social change would be a more effective response to their problems. In other cases, the side effects or other costs of cure may be more problematic than the illness or impairment itself. For example, people with mental illness have long documented the negative impacts of pharmaceuticals which reduce mood swings, but lead to lethargy and other negative symptoms. Cochlear implants sometimes cause complications, including potentially lethal infections such as meningitis. Limb-lengthening is a very stressful procedure causing considerable pain, frequent infections around the sites where pins are inserted into bones, and confinement to a wheelchair for many months. Even preventative medicine such as immunisation, while benefiting the vast majority, causes major impairment in a tiny proportion of those to whom it is administered.

However, the major practical problem with the cure agenda is the way that new medical research findings are associated with hyperbole and raised expectations, which then do not translate into benefits. This is a common theme in disability studies and disability activist reactions to medical research and media reports of cures. Sociologists of science and medicine have also drawn attention to the cycles of hype and disappointment around the new genetics (Smart, 2003) and other pioneering research such as xenotransplantation (Brown and Michael, 2003) and gene therapy (Stockdale 1999, Martin, 1999). For example, in the early 1990s there was considerable scientific excitement about gene therapy (Stockdale, 1999: 82; Orkin and Motulsky, 1995). The discovery of the CFTR gene, a mutation which causes cystic fibrosis, led the medical director of the US Cystic Fibrosis Foundation to say, 'We're not talking decades, we're talking years, a few years.' But still there are no cures in prospect – while there have been therapies and treatments which have alleviated the condition (Littlewood, 2004), it is still incurable. As one commentator said, 'These representations have consequences for people living with CF. They can give a false sense of hope, distress parents, and alienate adults with the disease' (Stockdale, 1999: 87).

The pursuit of cure has a long history, pre-dating genetic or stem cell research. For example, the spinal cord injury community have been discussing the prospects for cure since the 1950s, as Nicholas Watson has noted, such as this example of optimism from 1959:

> In the past twelve months paraplegia has been dealt some serious blows. Paraplegia has been attacked from all four sides this year . . . The four attackers: PVE, NPF, PN and the medical researchers . . . Medical science has come up with some advances too. Researchers have been able to repair damaged cords in animals and get nerve impulses past the break . . . A new substance to grow spinal nerves has been developed by Walter Reed scientists.
>
> (*Paraplegia News*, 1959: 2)

This extract comes from an editorial entitled 'Kick him while he's down'. Writing in *Paraplegia News* five years later, James Smittkamp is more realistic about the prospects:

> Twenty years ago the medical profession was almost unanimous in its belief that a cure was impossible. While this is still the majority view, some doubt of the old dogma has crept in and a few doctors now believe a cure can be found. But it will require considerable investment of talent, energy, money and time. From this reasoning two specific goals emerge: the elimination of paraplegia by finding a cure, and the alleviation of paraplegia until a cure can be found. Taking first the search for a cure, our problem is to determine the most promising approach . . . the obvious answer is specific research. Since

most doctors still consider a cure impossible, we must go to those few believers who still believe that 'all things are possible.'

(Smittkamp, 1964: 6)

This quotation shows that the impetus behind cure rhetoric often comes from people with the conditions and their families, not just from the scientific or medical community. These historical quotations also suggest that contemporary headlines such as 'Human stem cells allow paralysed mice to walk again' (Sample, 2005) should be treated very cautiously.

Representing people living with genetic conditions or other impairments as desperate for the cure can be a powerful way of drawing public attention to the condition, and levering charitable or governmental funding, as Nik Brown (2003) argues – 'the telling of sickness narratives in the context of technological promotion is a powerful means of creating research space, attractive investment and justifying morally challenging research' (Brown, 2003: 8). Brown talks about hope as part of 'dynamics of expectation' and discusses patient group participation in lobbying and funding research – 'a simultaneously moral and corporeal form of engagement' – although his own research found that patient organisations are now more ambivalent or sceptical, having had hopes dashed; 'the welding together of painful pathological biography and the fate of a biotechnological promise takes place at enormous cost to those who, for however long, are persuaded to share in the hope' (Brown, 2003: 8).

Yet, while those who hype medical research should be criticised, there is also a danger for those in the disability rights community – or indeed deconstructive social scientists in general – if they appear to relish the failure of medical research. Often, disability activists and social commentators take on the role of realists and cynics. Yet surely it would be wonderful if gene therapy or stem cell therapy did turn out to be effective in curing impairments and illnesses. While it is too soon to talk of cure, it is also too early to dismiss the possible potential of these frontier sciences. The difficulty for non-scientist commentators is how to form a judgement as to when the hype is justified. For example, early 1990s hype gene therapy did not translate into benefits. Is the current debate about stem cell research to be judged as similarly misguided? Is stem cell research more promising than gene therapy was, or will it be another busted flush in five years' time? Nik Brown argues that 'Communities of promise are constantly presented with the difficulty of judging the veracity of future claims. And we engage with these processes of judging whilst knowing that things rarely turn out as expected' (Brown, 2003: 17).

Anthropologist Sarah Franklin claims that

it is a mistake to think we can somehow factor out the hype, the media, or the work of the imagination in assessing the promises or the risks of new technology. This is not going to be possible, now or in the future, because it is precisely the importance of imagining new possibilities that fundamentally defines the whole issue of the new genetics and society.

(Franklin, 2003: 123)

## Cultural representation of cure

To look a little closer at the cultural representation of cure, I will focus on the example of stem cell research, and in particular the death of the actor Christopher Reeve in 2004. Reeve, who had suffered a very several spinal cord injury after a fall from a horse, had been a leading international figurehead in the quest to cure spinal cord injury. Through his profile and contacts, he was able to raise a large amount of money, which was used to fund The Reeve-Irvine Research Center, the strapline for which is 'Finding the cure'. Reeve and his medical allies always argued that regenerating the spinal cord was an achievable goal. He was quoted as saying, 'The time is at hand for breakthroughs in one of mankind's most heartbreaking problems, one that until now has resisted solution' (www.reeve.uci. edu/infodev.html).

Many disability rights activists disliked what Reeve stood for. He was seen as being unrealistic, as giving false hope, and as unrepresentative of disabled people. For example, he reportedly spent £270,000 on treatment and therapy each year, had eleven attendents, and benefited from donated equipment. He thus had privileges and opportunities unavailable to any other disabled person. Moreover, Reeve almost exclusively campaigned for medical research, rather than for disability rights. He could be dismissive of disabled people who didn't share his obsession with cure, and believe it was wrong to accommodate or come to terms with impairment. For these reasons, while some disabled people derived hope and inspiration from him, others rejected his work, the way he was represented, and even saw him as a traitor.

I examined coverage of Christopher Reeve's death in *The Times*, *The Independent*, the *Guardian*, *The Daily Telegraph* and the *Daily Mail* on 11 October 2004. Across the five newspapers sampled, there were twenty-four separate news stories, features, leading articles, op-ed pieces and obituaries. Coverage was dominated by words such as inspirational, indominitable, heroic, inspiring. *The Times*' treatment was typical: the front page news item was headlined:

'The all-American hero whose battle with disability gave hope to millions.'

The obituary described him as 'tirelessly campaigning for the disabled and their rights', a far from accurate description. A leading article saw Reeve as 'a source of inspiration for many who have been confronted by disability'. The *Guardian* leader writer reported that '[Reeve] subsequently became a role model for disabled people in the way he refused to allow the condition to conquer his spirit as well as his body, and for the tireless way he campaigned on disability issues'. As I argue in this chapter, the actual response of disabled people was more complex than this suggests.

Perhaps it is unreasonable to expect balance after someone has died. Yet critical or balanced statements were conspicuous by their absence. For example, *The Times* leader mentioned that Reeve 'was criticised by some for encouraging expectations beyond science's ability to deliver', and there were brief references to pro-life opposition to embryonic stem cell work (as well as an opinion piece by Michael Gove expressing anxieties about embryo research). *The Times* was typical in quoting actors, scientists and one representative of a spinal research charity, all of whom were positive about Reeve's role and message.

A more critical scientist, Colin Blakemore, was quoted in *The Independent* and also wrote a more balanced piece for the *Daily Mail*. He wrote, 'It is absolutely wrong to raise false expectations about the speed with which medical research progresses, but it takes people like Reeve, with their commitment and their certainty that they will be cured, to carry it forward.' Blakemore highlighted the difficulties with stem cell research, and pointed out the simple fact that it was never going to have been possible for Reeve to have walked again. Jeremy Laurance in *The Independent* ('The truth about Superman's achievements') and Ian Sample in the *Guardian* ('Is this the future of medicine?') stressed the uncertainty around stem cell research, and the time it would take to achieve clinical applications.

It is very rare for disabled people themselves, particularly critical voices, to be quoted in stories about cure research (Shakespeare, 1999a). Goggin and Newell (2004) analysed 300 news and features items on stem cells from Australian print media between May–June 2002. Disabled people were very rarely quoted as authorities, with the exception of several first-hand testimonial to the desire for salvation from people such as Christopher Reeve himself. Even a critical social analysis of different voices in the stem cell debate neglects disability rights perspectives (Ganchoff, 2004).

In the aftermath of Reeve's death, only two identified disabled people were quoted in the newspapers which I looked at. The *Guardian* quoted *Washington Post* columnist Charles Krauthammer (a wheelchair user) who called Reeve's public pronouncements 'disgracefully misleading', but in the context of a piece which concluded with a hope message and was entitled 'Life and death of a hero'. In the same newspaper, there was a piece by a spinal cord injured man explaining opposition from people with SCI and spinal injury units:

> Reeve was a controversial figure among people with spinal injuries and particularly with the more traditional medical establishments of spinal injury units. His message of hope for a cure was regarded as irresponsible and misleading. Whenever his name was mentioned it was either with frustration or a sneer, and I have often heard it said: 'His name is a dirty word in this house.'

However, the author's own views were very positive about Reeve and cure.

While the mainstream media were very positive about Reeve, the same cannot be said for the disability press. For example, activist Tara Flood was quoted in *Disability Now* as saying that Reeve 'Clearly surrounded himself with people who made him believe a cure was just around the corner' when it was 'potentially generations away . . . He was in a position where he could have done huge amounts for disabled people but chose a different route.'

Bill Albert argued that the problem was that Reeve saw his disability as a medical issue. However, *Disability Now* did include one dissenting voice from the Spinal Injuries Association, which was more positive about Reeve's work. Online, BBC websites recorded many testimonies from disabled people and others which were very positive about Reeve, with phrases such as 'Reeve was inspirational figure' and 'Reeve changed how I look at life'. No quotations from disabled people who opposed Reeve were featured. Certainly, disability rights contributors to online discussion groups such as the international disability-research list were largely negative about Reeve, and when I wrote a more balanced column on the BBC Disability website, I received very negative feedback from the radical community.

Studying media coverage of embryonic stem cell research in 2000, Clare Williams *et al.* (2003) found that there were five TV news bulletins which featured patients or patient support groups speaking in favour of stem cell research, and no examples of them speaking against (out of a total of eight bulletins). Only Labour MPs featured as often in bulletins. They also found that twenty-two newspaper articles featured supportive scientists and doctors, while four featured supportive patients or patient groups, and none featured critical patients or patient support groups. The views of both disability rights groups and women's voices were marginalised in coverage. As I have shown, the same is true of coverage of Reeve's death.

Yet it would be wrong to assume that the disability community has a single or coherent view of people like Christopher Reeve, or stem cell research more generally. While mainstream media may have been dominated by non-disabled pro-research voices, ordinary disabled people did write in to support Reeve's work. Other research finds patient activists in favour of stem cell and other medical advances (Ganchoff, 2004). Moreover, disability activist and disability studies debates are skewed towards anti-cure, anti-Reeve voices.

## Difficult cases

Examination of media coverage and lay voices shows the importance of capturing the complexity and variation in disability responses. Looking more closely at a few case studies of cures and therapies shows the need for nuance in judgement. The Hastings Center volume *Surgically Shaping Children* (Parens, 2006) provides just such a pluralist and carefully argued account of three sorts of therapy decisions: correction of cleft lip and palate; gender reassignment surgery; and limb-lengthening in children with restricted growth. As the author shows, such cases are complex, because the patients involved are often too young to choose freely for themselves: parents have to make difficult decisions in what they believe to be the best interests of the child. This brings into conflict two values at the heart of parenting: to support the well-being of our chilren, and to let them unfold in their own way. The contributors to the Hastings Center volume broadly agreed with parents deciding on early surgery to repair cleft lip and palate; opposed parents deciding on behalf of their children when it comes to intersex surgery; and believed that children themselves should be supported to make decisions about limb-lengthening.

One problem of the Hastings Center approach (and of previous research in this area by Priscilla Alderson, 1993) is that there is a risk of individualising the treatment decision. In other words, while I support the involvement of children in decisions about their treatment, there is a risk of both children and adults being influenced by a wider cultural climate in the direction of accepting normalisation. For example, I think it possible that children who consent to limb-lengthening may be implicitly influenced by their non-disabled parents' desires, as well as by the broader cultural messages in wider society. Limb-lengthening decisions are taken in the early teenage years, a period of the life course when pressure towards, and desire for, social conformity is at its height. Evidence that those who have undertaken the surgery are glad that they have done so is also problematic: after so great an investment of time and endurance of pain, and with a changed body shape, it is hard for any individual then to admit it may have been a mistake, or to say that they are not happy with the result.

One of the more controversial forms of cure is use of cochlear implants to correct hearing impairment. This has been opposed by Deaf people, who challenge the impairment-based definition of deafness. To Deaf activists, being Deaf is about being a cultural minority, not being disabled. Deafness becomes a cultural identity based on shared language, like a minority ethnic community. For this reason, Deaf people often refuse to identify with disabled people, whom they regard as having impairments. Deaf people usually welcome the birth of deaf children, who can then be enculturated into Deaf culture, through the use of sign language. Recently, there was also the controversial case of a Deaf lesbian couple who took active steps to maximise the chances of their child being deaf by choosing a Deaf sperm donor.

There seem to be internal contradictions in the Deaf approach to cochlear implants. First, if Deafness is really nothing to do with impairment, then logically there would be no reason for Deaf people to oppose impairment reduction. Second, if Deafness is about being a member of a sign language community, there is nothing to stop hearing children of Deaf adults being members of that community too: indeed, there is a thriving Children of Deaf Adults (CODA) movement which enjoys membership in both Deaf and hearing worlds.

Third, the vast majority of deaf children are born to hearing adults. Because their parents are not native signers, it would not be easy for these children to become native sign language users. For them, the best option may be to maximise speech and hearing through cochlear implants, so that they can have a chance of communicating with their parents and joining the hearing world. The dilemma for deaf children of Deaf adults is that the maximum benefit of a cochlear implant comes when the child forgoes sign language and concentrates entirely on learning to speak and hear and lip read. Therefore if Deaf parents implant their deaf child, they are sacrificing their best hope of communicating effectively with their own child, who will additionally suffer from having parents whose speech is probably limited. For this reason, the opposition of Deaf parents to implanting their own children is understandable, but should not prevent hearing parents using this technology to improve the life chances of their deaf child.

A difficult case is presented by autism and other forms of 'neuro-diversity' (Happé,1994; Hodge, 2005). In recent years, partly due to the development of internet-based forms of communication, a community of people with autism, Asperger's syndrome and related conditions have challenged the devaluing and pathologisation of these experiences. From a 'Neuro Diverse' perspective, different ways of thinking and relating are not impairments, but just differences. A more flexible society would be able to accommodate neuro-diverse people, and value their strengths and aptitudes, rather than seeking to prevent or cure these conditions.

While not dismissing this approach, it should be noted that many people on the autistic spectrum do have significant problems arising from their cognitive differences. They may have severe learning difficulties; they may have extreme difficulties relating to other people or participating in society; unlike dominant media representations, they may have no compensating skills or aptitudes. In other words, those people with high functioning autism or Asperger's syndrome who talk of autism as an alternative style may not be representative of others with the condition. While it is always valuable to promote acceptance and an understanding of difference, many families would welcome prevention, therapy or cure of autism (Kelly, 2005). The case of autistic spectrum conditions is a reminder of two important features of impairment highlighted in previous chapters. First, there is a hierachy of impairment: different impairments have different impacts, and the same impairment can have different effects. Second, mild to moderate impairment may not be a difficulty for anyone, given supportive and flexible environments prepared to respect and value difference. However, severe forms of impairment will often cause considerable problems and limitations and sometimes suffering and distress for the individual and their families. The goal of promoting cultural respect and social acceptance for people with impairment should not distract us from the importance of mitigating or preventing impairment via individual medical or psychological therapies.

## Conclusion

In this chapter I have argued for a more balanced approach to cure and therapy within disability studies. From a critical realist perspective, committed to understanding the operation of disability on different ontological levels, biomedical and psychological intervention has an important role. It would be foolish to hope for quick results from stem cell or gene therapy research. It would be dangerous to rely on medical research as an alternative to barrier removal. However, if safe, effective treatments eventually materialise then disabled people will benefit and quality of life will improve. Resort to medicine is not contrary to other objectives of disability rights, and activists and scholars should be critical supporters of the endeavour to mitigate or prevent impairment.

However, a wise approach to the issue would also recognise the ubiquity of impairment. Medicine will never banish the problems and limitations of embodiment. As argued previously, impairment is a predicament which faces everyone, in some form and at some time. The ambition to minimise illness and impairment should be balanced with the need to accept limitations, and find ways of living with them. Denigrating or misrepresenting the lives of existing disabled people in the search for cures, even with the noble aim of raising funds for research, cannot be justified. Obsession with normality and perfection, ultimately unattainable or false goals, is harmful to well-being and self-esteem (Martz, 2001).

Biomedical research is not the only way to enhance the life of disabled people, either in Britain or globally. In fact, taking an international perspective reveals that there are more pressing disabling conditions than the rare disorders or late onset conditions for which stem cell research and genetics may eventually bring benefits (Shakespeare, 2005b). The majority of the world's citizens are still impaired by preventable diseases such as malaria or TB, or other socially caused conditions arising from accidents, malnutrition, poverty and war. Ninety per cent of the world's pharmaceutical research is conducted on diseases which affect 10 per cent of the world's population (Flory and Kitcher, 2004). As Philip Kitcher argues, 'When millions of children die every year from malaria, how can we justify our expenditures on research into Lesch-Nyhan syndrome, cystic fibrosis, even the common forms of cancer?' (Kitcher, 1997: 324).

Another interesting feature of contemporary biomedical research is that while most projects are directed at ameliorating impairment and illness, new products and techniques find wider application in non-disabled populations (Juengst, 1998). Examples such as Viagra , human growth hormone (Conrad and Potter, 2004) and Prozac (Elliot, 1999) show how difficult it is to police the line between therapies and enhancement (Buchanan *et al.*, 2000: 118). Jackie Scully and Christoph Rehmann-Sutter (2001) argue that the use of the therapy/enhancement distinction further reinforces the pathologisation of impairment and people with impairment. They argue that attention should be paid to the consequences of concrete intervention, rather than reliance on a simplistic distinction to validate/invalidate therapeutic approaches. While the therapy/enhancement debate is beyond the scope of this chapter, it is important because it suggests that rather than equalising the natural lottery – creating greater equality by compensating and correcting impairments which render people disadvantaged – some biotechnologies may ultimately increase inequality, because they enable those who are non-disabled to further enhance their capabilities, leaving the impaired at a greater comparative disadvantage.

While these points, cautions and concerns are important – and have been well made by many bioethicists and some disability studies commentators – they do not provide intrinsic objections to pursuing medical research, alongside other strategies. But they do suggest that there are pressing questions for wider social regulation and debate, in order that the coming applications of biomedicine should be exploited to benefit the many, rather than the few, and to enhance, rather than to exploit and divide. We require what Flory and Kitcher (2004: 59) define as 'well-ordered science', where the voices of those directly affected are heard, where research is directed towards those questions which are most significant, and where scientists take their moral obligations seriously.

# Chapter 8

# Autonomy at the end of life

Disability issues in bioethics are highly contested because they bring up powerful emotional issues: questions about the permissability of technological intervention; the vulnerability of disabled people; the widespread non-disabled perception that impairment is a fate worse than death; the historical backdrop of abuse, oppression and murder. These factors are common to debates at both the beginning of life, and the end of life. Fears about eugenics and about euthanasia form the substrate of the disability rights response to bioethical arguments about autonomy and the value of life (Asch, 2001).

End of life questions are poignant, first because they seem to threaten the very existence of disabled people, even more personally and directly than questions about prenatal diagnosis. Second, if individuals are permitted to end their life on the grounds of suffering and restriction, this potentially sends a message that impairment is so awful that no one would want to go on living in such a state. Third, a narrow focus on impairment and suffering again risks obscuring the social-contexts which often determine the quality of disabled people's lives, in particular the availability of independent living and civil rights protections from exclusion and discrimination.

In recent years, the end of life debate has assumed a high profile in many western countries. The US state of Oregon legalized assisted sucide in 1997; the Netherlands legalized euthanasia and assisted suicide in 2002, after a thirty-year period of non-prosecution of such cases; Belgium legalized euthanasia in 2002 (Finlay *et al.*, 2005). In Britain there has been a string of high-profile legal cases such as those of Miss B, a disabled woman who wished for her ventilator to be turned off so that she could die, rather than live in an impaired state; Diane Pretty, a woman terminally ill with motor neurone disease who petitioned for her partner to be able to assist her to commit suicide; and Reginald Crewe and other terminally ill individuals who have sought to travel to Switzerland where the voluntary organisation Dignitas offers an assisted suicide service. Partly in response to such cases, Lord Joffe has introduced several bills into the House of Lords to permit assisted suicide in Britain, supported by the Voluntary Euthanasia Society (Epstein, 2005). In the United States, there was huge public interest in the case of Terry Schiavo, a brain damaged woman whose former husband petitioned for her life-support system to be switched off, against the wishes of her parents and 'Pro-Life' campaigners. Assisted suicide has also been the subject of the high-profile and award winning films *The Sea Inside* (Dir. Amenabar, 2004) and *Million Dollar Baby* (Dir. Eastwood, 2004). This unprecedented coverage of end of life issues perhaps contributes to the perception and fear amongst disabled people that their lives are in danger.

Notwithstanding the validity of these concerns, it is important to note that the passionate debate about disability rights at the end of life also bolsters an identity politics approach. Organisations such as Not Dead Yet, high-profile battles against euthanasia enthusiasts such as Kevorkian, and emotive comparisons with Nazi euthanasia all fuel a plot narrative which variously suggests that other family members, doctors, or society desire the death of disabled people. Such a victim position is potent in raising the profile of the disability rights movement, and bolstering disability identity (for example Darke, 2004). The potent image of vulnerable disabled people is also encouraged by the vociferous 'Pro-Life' movement which uses an alliance with disabled campaigners to back its opposition to choice, at both the beginning and end of life.

Typically, the discourse of disability rights opposition operates at the level of generality, rather than specifics: interventions are usually emotive and rhetorical, rather than rational and analytical; individuals are denounced; diverse issues are conflated. The disability rights critique obscures the range of issues at the end of life. These include decisions about reuscitation (cardio-pulmonary reuscitation, or CPR); advance directives and living wills; withdrawal of treatment; assisted suicide; voluntary euthanasia; non-voluntary euthanasia. Each raises different questions, and a careful response should differentiate between them, even though they all raise questions about the death of people who may be defined as disabled.

In particular, it is important to distinguish situations where the autonomy of disabled people is undermined (abuse of 'do not resuscitate' notices, non-voluntary euthanasia) from situations where disabled or terminally ill people themselves are exercising their autonomy by requesting assistance with death, or withdrawal of treatment (advance directives, assisted suicide). A failure to draw relevant distinctions and a failure to engage with the clinical realities undermines many disability rights critiques. As an example of the complexities of what appears to be a straightforward end of life issue, I will turn briefly to the DNR ('do not resuscitate') controversy.

The background to this controversy lies in instances when disabled or elderly people have gone into hospital, often for minor operations, and discovered that a clinician has scribbled 'DNR' on their chart, without consultation. To the patient, this can be very distressing. It appears that a judgement has been made that the patient's life is not worth preserving, and that clinicians are unfairly discriminating between disabled and non-disabled people. Emotive claims – 'the NHS is killing disabled people' – express the outrage of the disability movement, and spread fear among disabled people who use hospitals.

Sometimes, fears of discrimination and prejudice may be justified. There are also fears that patients given DNR orders receive poorer treatment (Mohammed *et al.*, 2005). And it is certainly the case that decisions about cardio-pulmonary resuscitation (CPR) should always involve discussion with the patient and their relatives, which is a central element in the good practice statement agreed by the UK Resuscitation Council and doctors and nurses organisations (Resuscitation Council, 2001). However, while there have been abuses, claims such as 'the NHS is killing disabled people' seem exaggerated.

Furthermore, CPR may not always be the straightforward benefit which it appears. It is likely that the general public has an exaggerated view of the efficacy of attempts at resuscitation. Even professionals regularly over-estimate the possibilities of CPR being successful (Wagg *et al.*, 1995). Most lay people's experience of CPR comes via medical soap operas such as ER. On television, CPR has a very high success rate. One study of television representation showed short-term survival (one hour) after resuscitation in 75 per cent of cases (Diem *et al.*, 1996). By contrast, 40 per cent short-term success is accepted to be the upper limit in practice, and most sources give a figure of 25 per cent of patients being successfully rescuscitated in the short term. The same TV study found 67 per cent of CPR cases survived until discharge from hospital. By contrast, a range of studies of long-term survival have produced figures of 2–30 per cent for those experiencing cardiac arrest outside a hospital, and 6.5–15 per cent for those experiencing arrest while in hospital. For elderly patients, it is suggested a figure of 5 per cent long-term survival after CPR would be more realistic. Unrealistic media portrayal, therefore, reinforces the perception that CPR is a miraculous intervention with a high chance of success. For this reason, many clinicians prefer the acronym 'DNAR' to clarify that the decisions is 'do not attempt resuscitation'.

Not only does CPR not succeed in the majority of cases, but it can also cause harm to patients. CPR involves: checking that airways are clear, and sometimes inserting a tube into the mouth and airway; air or oxygen being pumped into the lungs; vigorous repeated pressure on the chest to pump blood to the brain and other vital organs until normal heartbeat is restored; it may include the use of an electric shock (defibrillation) to restart the heart. CPR is often a distressing experience for patients, relatives and staff. There are some disabled or elderly people for whom CPR could be hugely traumatic or sometimes even lethal. For example, people with osteoporosis or osteogenesis imperfecta have fragile bones, which could be damaged if clinicians attempted to restart their heart, resulting in fractured sternum or ribcage and possibly lacerated lungs. The outcome would either be a much more painful death at the time, or temporary survival in a state of extreme discomfort. For the rest of the minority who survive CPR, research shows that 20–50 per cent suffer neurological impairment, ranging from slight brain damage to persistent vegetative state (Mohr and Kettler, 1997). In other words, choosing to decline CPR may be a rational choice, given the realities:

> If CPR were a benign, risk-free procedure that offered a good hope of long-term survival in the face of otherwise certain death, few people would ever

choose to have medical personnel withhold resuscitation. But controversy surrounds the use of CPR precisely because the procedure can lead to prolonged suffering, severe neurologic damage, or an undignified death.

(Diem *et al.*, 1996: 1581)

For the same reasons, doctors may think CPR contra-indicated in such cases and suggest DNAR.

The evidence shows that if CPR procedure and outcome evidence is properly explained to patients, they are more likely to decline resuscitation and to request DNAR notices. For example, in one study, 41 per cent of acute patients initially opted for CPR. When informed of the evidence about efficacy and outcome, 22 per cent opted for CPR. In a group of people with chronic illness whose life expectancy was less than a year, only 11 per cent initially opted for CPR. After being informed of the evidence, only 5 per cent opted for CPR (Cherniack, 2002: 303). Of course, an alternative way of interpreting these findings is that those who explain CPR and DNAR to patients are doing so in ways which encourage or even subtly coerce people into adopting an approach which clinicians themselves approve of.

Abuse of DNAR must be exposed and opposed. Moroever, DNAR should not trigger diminished quality of care (Mohammed *et al.*, 2005). Yet, properly used, DNAR notices have a place in medicine. There has been a transition from medical paternalism to a partnership model in DNAR guidelines. DNAR notices are used in a minority of cases, and the abuse of DNAR is rarer still. All medical decisions should be based on consultation between professionals and patients, although doctors have to use their professional judgement as to whether a course of action will be clinically effective and in the patient's best interest. Equally, it may be rational for a patient to request a DNAR notice. Everyone, disabled or not, has an interest in having a good death, and CPR is often painful, undignified and futile. The conclusion I draw from the CPR/DNAR debate is that calm and evidence-based deliberation is usually more useful to disabled people than extreme rhetoric.

My position on end of life, as will become evident in this chapter, is based on consistent support for the choices and desires of disabled people themselves, not on disability rights ideology. For most of the time, the disability rights movement supports the autonomy of disabled people. The slogan 'choices and rights' has been an important rallying cry in many life domains. For example, autonomy is the basis of independent living philosophy, which campaigns for disabled people to have control over their own lives. It seems to me to be inconsistent to support autonomy for disabled people in all matters except the moment and manner of their death. The remainder of this chapter will focus on the assisted suicide debate, in order to analyse these general issues within a particular and topical context.

## Assisted suicide and disability rights opposition

The most famous disability rights group campaigning against assisted suicide is the US Not Dead Yet, founded in opposition to Dr Jack Kevorkian, the former physician who encouraged 130 ill or disabled people to die by offering his services. Their strapline is 'the resistance' and their website argues, 'Though often described as compassionate, legalized medical killing is really about a deadly double standard for people with severe disabilities, including both conditions that are labeled terminal and those that are not.' Not Dead Yet sees assisted suicide as giving medical professionals immunity from killing disabled people. Founder Diane Coleman argues that economic pressures within the private healthcare system, together with lack of protection within the courts, would threaten disabled people if assisted suicide was legalised in the United States.

Most US disability rights activists and disability studies academics appear to support the position taken by Not Dead Yet (for example Gill, 1992, 2000; Silvers, 1998). For example, the historian Paul Longmore (2003) has written eloquently on the Elizabeth Bouvia case, and has argued that assisted suicide activists have a much broader agenda than the right to die in terminal illness, seeking to extend coverage to all disabled people. Adrienne Asch takes a position in support of Not Dead Yet in her account of bioethics and disability (2001). However, a few writers on disability (for example Batavia, 1997) have adopted positions in support of autonomy.

In the UK, disability rights opposition to assisted suicide was prompted by the House of Lords Bill to legalise assisted suicide introduced by Lord Joffe in 2004 and 2005. Joffe would have mandated physician assisted suicide in a very narrow set of cases. An individual would only be able to take advantage of the provision if (1) she was terminally ill, and expected to die naturally within a short period and (2) she was suffering unbearably. The Bill thus extended to disabled people the power to end their lives – which non-disabled people are able to do through a decision to commit suicide – as well as ensuring that doctors would be able to give assistance and advice to terminally ill people so that the appropriate drugs to ensure successful and pain-free suicide were made available and used effectively.

Organisations in the UK disability movement have been almost unanimous in their opposition to the Joffe Bill, as were the majority of disability rights academics and activists. In 2004, I submitted evidence and appeared as a witness in favour of the Bill, but to my knowledge was the only prominent voice from the disability movement who spoke out in favour of assisted suicide. Due to the 2005 election, this version of the Bill failed. When Lord Joffe reintroduced his Assisted Dying Bill in November 2005, the *Disability Now* newspaper again printed a selection of prominent disabled people's views: thirteen argued against the Bill, four argued in favour. Meanwhile, the majority of respondents to the *Disability Now* November 2005 poll argued in favour. Given that the Joffe Bill appeared to promote the autonomy of disabled people, ensuring the right to a good death, and not undermining the possibility of a good life, why did the leaders of the disability movement, almost without exception, oppose it?

One class of fears centres on the environment in which people make decisions. Disabled people may be vulnerable to different pressures, which in practice under-mine the possibility of them making an autonomous decision. For example, in the immediate context, direct pressure may be be exerted on disabled people to end their lives against their will. Healthcare systems and relatives may want to save the costs of supporting a dying person for many months. There are historical and contemporary precedents for so-called 'mercy killing', and there are fears that disabled people will be pressured by relatives or professionals to request assisted suicide.

More generally, the wider cultural context may also influence disabled people. Decisions are always made in a social context. Campaigns for assisted suicide and voluntary euthanasia have sometimes emphasised the pain, humiliation and difficulty of disability in ways which are derogatory to disabled people, and cause fear and alarm in non-disabled people (Hurst, n.d.). Similarly, most people are afraid of dying and of death. Davis comments, 'The phrase "death with dignity" is very often used to mean the deliberately procured death of an ill or disabled person, and strongly implies that vulnerable people are only "dignified" in death' (Davis, 2004: 1).Exaggerating the difficulties and suffering of impairment-related death – and ignoring the success of palliative care – will distort people's reactions and perhaps stimulate demand for assisted suicide.

Making assisted suicide available might also send an implicit message that it is logical and desirable for disabled people to end their own lives, or that disabled people's lives are inferior to those of non-disabled people (Campbell, 2003). This cultural belief may influence the attitudes of people who live and work with disabled people. These messages and attitudes in turn might feed back into disabled people's own views about their actions and choices, making it more likely that they will choose assisted suicide, even if it is against their best interests and they would not freely have taken that step in the absence of influence.

Many disabled people feel vulnerable and depressed from time to time, particularly after first diagnosis of impairment or chronic illness. Living with both impairment and disability is not easy. Many disabled people have at different points wanted to end their lives. With support and over time, most disabled people have come to terms with their impairments and learned to accommodate to their restrictions, reporting a good quality of life and no longer wishing to end their own lives. Disabled opponents of assisted suicide, many of whom have gone through this trajectory themselves, fear that other disabled people may make irreversible decisions, soon after onset of impairment, and deny themselves the possibility of living a better life as a disabled person in future.

There may also be an impact on people who are not currently disabled, but may be anxious about becoming impaired. Fear of impairment is widespread among non-disabled people who are unfamiliar with disabled people. Research has shown considerable cultural prejudice against disabled people and a commonly expressed belief that it would be better to be dead than disabled. These fears need to be challenged, and the positive aspects and contributions of disabled people need to be emphasised. Impairment and disability are part of the human condition, and society needs to come to terms with disability, not encourage people to think that disabled lives are not worth living.

Of course, the influences on a person's decisions to seek assisted suicide can be material, as well as cultural and attitudinal. If the full range of independent living options (housing, technology, assistance, etc.) are not available, then the lives of people with impairments and terminal illnesses will seem harder and they may be more likely to opt to end their life. The disability movement has argued that a person must have had access to the full range of care and independent living possibilities, prior to being entitled to request assisted suicide. Equally, the hospice movement provides evidence that palliative care and pain relief can ease dying. The availability of palliative care and of hospice care is very important. A person must have had access to these facilities, prior to being entitled to request assisted suicide. In countries like the Netherlands, where voluntary euthanasia is an established practice, the hospice movement and palliative care has not developed to the same degree as in UK.

Second, there is a set of questions about those who may be entitled to have an assisted suicide request honoured. 'Unbearable suffering' has been presented as a qualification for assisted suicide. But how should this be defined? It is almost impossible to agree an objective measure of pain and suffering, and everyone reacts to impairment and illness differently. Not everyone finds a particular level of pain or restriction unbearably awful. Many disabled people are living with the pain and dependency, technological and physical, which is cited as evidence for the rationality of a decision by others to seek assisted suicide. For example, many disabled people are tube-fed throughout their lives, yet tube-feeding for some assisted suicide advocates marks a stage of terminal illness when death would be appropriate and desirable. For example, Ed Roberts, an influential US disability activist, said:

> I've been on a respirator for twenty-six years, and I watch these people's cases. They're just as dependent on a respirator as I am. The major difference is that they know they're going to be forced to live in a nursing home – or they're already there – and I'm leading a quality of life. That's the only difference. It's not the respirator. It's the money.
>
> (quoted in Priestley, 2004: 174)

Disabled people living with tube feeding, or ventilation, or other forms of high dependency fear that their own lives will be devalued, or may even be at risk, as a result of the decisions or attitudes of others who do not want to live in such conditions.

Another qualification often cited is 'terminal illness'. But again, it is not clear how to define this state. Many disabled people live throughout their lives with conditions which are defined as terminal. For example, impairments such as cystic fibrosis, muscular dystrophy, multiple sclerosis, HIV/AIDS are all currently incurable, and generally result in premature death. Some people who are diagnosed with these conditions decide that life is no longer worth living, even though they are currently not severely impaired. Would people with such impairments be considered terminally ill, and hence candidates for assisted suicide? Moroever, many of these illnesses have an episodic and fluctuating presentation: individuals may develop complications, enter a critical phase and appear on the verge of death, but with appropriate medical care may recover to live on for many more years. Only in retrospect is it clear when the terminal phase of terminal illness has begun.

Even though the Joffe Bill was restricted to people with terminal illnesses who were likely to die within a short period, many disability campaigners feared that it would be easy to extend the rights or cultural expectation of assisted suicide to disabled people in general, not just people who are in the terminal stage of a terminal illness. The fear of a slippery slope underpins both the contextual and the categorical arguments. If limited and careful assisted suicide legislation – such as the Joffe Bill – were approved, disability rights campaigners fear that the process would not stop there. They suggest the following narrative might unfold: the safe-guards to ensure autonomous decision making would be weakened, as legalisation made it more acceptable, and people began to feel pressurised to opt for death. The category of people who had the right to assisted suicide could be extended, to include those who are not in the terminal stages of incurable illness and in unbearable suffering, and also many people who are currently living with impair-ment, restriction and discomfort. By degrees, policy might be broadened until assisted suicide turned into voluntary euthanasia, and then voluntary euthanasia became non-voluntary euthanasia.

The third objection suggests that assisted suicide legalisation would be a form of unfair discrimination. For example, central to the Not Dead Yet case is that assisted suicide provisions violate equal protection under the Americans with Disabilities Act, because while non-disabled people would be prevented or discouraged from committing sucide, people with terminal illness – who are disabled people – would be permitted or encouraged to do so: legalised assisted suicide, in this reading, would legitimate disability discrimination.

A final objection, made eloquently for example by Alison Davis (2004), is the claim that life is an inalienable right. This means that life is a right of which you cannot be deprived, not even by yourself. According to this perspective, even if a majority of the public, including a majority of disabled people support assisted suicide, it would still be wrong. Even if there was no evidence of abuse or coercion whatsoever, it should remain prohibited. Yet the idea that life is inalienable seems to be an a priori assumption. It is usually rooted in religious prohibitions. There seems to be no clear reason why those who do not adopt a theological approach to morality should accept the concept.

## The autonomy argument for assisted suicide

The most powerful argument for permitting assisted suicide arises from the principle of autonomy (Woods, 2002, 2005). Within liberal democracies, people are usually entitled to choices as to how to live their lives, even if these choices conflict with the values of others, so long as their actions do not harm others. In other words, although I may not want to end my own life, neither I nor the state should prevent others taking this step. Control over one's own body is one of the most important of rights, and restricting someone's ability to choose how and when to die is regarded by many as intrusive.

Choice is a very important principle for the disability movement. For example, disability rights campaigners have fought for independent living, meaning the right to choose where and how to live and be supported. Where a person cannot carry out physical tasks, the principles of independent living suggests that she should be able to employ others to carry out those tasks, under her control (Morris, 1993a). Similarly, disability rights campaigners have fought for choices freely to express sexuality, to form relationships and reproduce, with assistance where necessary (Shakespeare *et al.*, 1996; Earle, 1999). Autonomy in healthcare is an important dimension of the choices and rights at the centre of disability movement ideology. For example, people should be free from unwanted treatment, and should be consulted in decisions which affect them.

It is therefore paradoxical and appears inconsistent that the disability movement should support freedom of choice in every area of life except the desire of a disabled person to end their life. Moreover, providing assistance to commit suicide could be said to empower a disabled person to realise their desires, in the same way as assistance in other activities. In law, people who are dependent on life-sustaining treatment already have the right to request withdrawal of treatment (for example, having their ventilator switched off, as Miss B requested). But those who are not treatment dependent have no such possibility of ending their life. A disabled person might be unable to commit suicide, due to their physical situation, whereas a non-disabled person could carry through their wishes and take steps to bring about their own death: attempting suicide is no longer illegal in Britain. For example, Diane Pretty complained that she was physically incapable of killing herself without assistance, and needed her partner to help her die. Supporting her claim, Liberty, the human rights group, argued that she should have the same rights to kill herself as anyone else (Priestley, 2004: 173). Giving disabled people assistance to die would therefore remove an inequality, putting them in the same position as a non-disabled person. Logically, this seems a reasonable extension of the principles of autonomy, independent living and non-discrimination.

Moreover, the arguments of disability rights campaigners who oppose assisted suicide are themselves framed in the language of autonomy: it is claimed that if some people were to exercise their choice to commit suicide, this would infringe or undermine the choices of others not to commit suicide (Campbell, 2003). Yet it is not clear, conceptually, how this follows. Different disabled people have different views and desires. The desires or decisions of one disabled person should not have direct implications for the desires or decisions of another disabled person. For example, if some disabled people want to use personal assistance services, this does not imply that everyone else should be forced to adopt the same approach to support and care.

Empirically, some disabled people want to exercise the right to die: the cases of Reginald Crew, Diane Pretty, Miss B and others are examples of this phenomenon. Moreover, survey evidence suggests that disability activists and advocates who oppose assisted suicide are in a minority among disabled people. When the Disability Rights Commission conducted an online survey in 2003, 63 per cent of respondents supported new laws on end of life. Polling conducted by MORI for the Voluntary Euthanasia Society in 2004 found that 80 per cent of disabled people supported the Joffe Bill to legalise assisted suicide in controlled circumstances. This data seems to suggest that not only is disability movement opposition to assisted suicide contradicting the important disability rights principle of autonomy, but also that disability rights advocates and organisations are not representative of the population whom they claim to speak for.

In some cases, society restricts liberty in order to protect people from the consequences of their actions. For example, in Britain it is compulsory to wear a seat belt in a car or crash helmet on a motorbike, even though the only person who might otherwise be put at risk is an individual capable of freely choosing to travel unprotected. Prohibition of drugs is another example of protecting vulnerable individuals from bad decisions in their own best interests. It may be argued that terminally ill people also need to be protected from the consequences of a mistaken choice. Yet the person who fails to wear a seatbelt or helmet or uses drugs has not decided that they want to die. They have been careless, or believed that the pleasurable sensations outweigh the medical risks, or taken a gamble that they will not be harmed. These are different cases to the situation of someone who has thought carefully about their predicament, and expressed a deliberate and continuing desire to end their life.

Alternatively, it could be said to be inconsistent to limit the right of disabled people to assisted suicide to cases of terminal illness. A fully consistent equality argument suggests that disabled people should be free to choose suicide at any time or for any reason, because this is a power which non-disabled people can exercise. Yet, there is a general presumption that suicide is to be prevented where possible. Even though suicide has been decriminalised, it is a moral duty for third parties to try to dissuade a person to commit suicide. Therefore it would not be right for society to help any disabled or non-disabled person to commit suicide on autonomy grounds. The only socially sanctioned case where suicide becomes a legitimate choice is in the case of end stage terminal illness. This is because having an end stage terminal illness is morally relevant to the decision to end life. The individual does not have the prospect of a continuing life or of recovery from illness. The person may be suffering pain and discomfort and restriction. While they are aware that they are dying, they do not know when death will come. Modern medical care can keep people alive, who would previously have died much more quickly. Dying people may have to endure days or even weeks of suffering, and witness their relatives and friends watching this extended process. Assisted suicide hastens death by a matter of days or possibly weeks.

In other words, choosing death can be rational for people in an end of life situation. The palliative care community largely oppose legalization of assisted suicide, because of a belief that good palliative care can ease all deaths (Finlay *et al.*, 2005). But even with palliative care, hospice facilities and support, some deaths are difficult and it is rational to fear them. Of course, assisted suicide is certainly not something which all terminally ill people will want. Some people cope better with restrictions, find value in enduring suffering, and find alternative sources of meaning and pleasure. They will want to extend their life as long as possible, because they want to spend time with loved ones, and experience every minute available to them. But others find the situation of prolonged dying unendurable and their suffering futile and unnecessary. Many patients want to control the circumstances of their death (Miller *et al.*, 2004). Views on end of life are highly personal, depending on religious and moral values, and an individual's capacity to cope with pain or restriction. One person's judgement does not have implications for another person's right to life or dignity or respect.

For the same reason, it is not discriminatory to distinguish between terminally ill people and non-disabled people. Justice demands treating like cases alike, and unlike cases differently. If all disabled people were given access to assisted suicide, just because they were disabled, this would be discrimination (Davis, 2004). In normal situations, having a different physical or mental state should not be relevant to the judgement of the legitimacy of ending life. But in the specific situation of a end stage terminal illness, where the individual is suffering greatly, there are morally relevant reasons to waive the usual prohibitions on suicide, and to enable patients to die painlessly and at a time of their own choosing.

## Pragmatic arguments about assisted suicide

As well as arguments about the legitimacy of choosing a 'good death', the importance of supporting autonomy, and the empirical evidence of disabled people's own wishes, there are also several pragmatic arguments for making assisted suicide legal.

As with abortion, if assisted suicide is illegal, it does not mean that it will not occur. Because many people have a strong desire to end their lives to avoid the suffering of a slow and painful death, people will take steps to bring this about. For example, individuals will attempt to travel to places where assisted suicide is permitted. This can lead to the complications, distress and difficulty of so-called 'death tourism', for example in the case of Reginald Crew and others. Alternatively, some people will attempt to end their lives without assistance. This 'underground assisted suicide' may lead to the dangers of botched suicide, and the risks of prosecution of assisters, fears of which may make a terminally ill person's situation more difficult and anxious (Magnusson, 2002). The analogy with backstreet abortion suggests that providing regulated and medically safe provision is better than driving the situation underground, putting people at further risk of harm and criminalising those who, often for good motives, seek to help people in need.

The second pragmatic argument is based on the suggestion that though a majority of people want to have access to assisted suicide, only a minority will ever choose to exercise their right to end their life (as data from Oregon and the Netherlands suggests). Knowing that assisted suicide is available may often reduce the anxiety of dying people. Fear of pain and other symptoms may be mitigated by the knowledge that there is another way out, if it all gets too much. The possibility of controlling death can be life-enhancing.

A national survey by Clive Seale (2006) reveals that, in some cases, British doctors already hasten the death of their patients in different ways. The data shows that physician-assisted deaths are very rare: none of his respondents had assisted the suicide of patients, and only 0.16 per cent had performed voluntary euthanasia and 0.33 per cent non-voluntary euthanasia. This suggests that the disability rights community's suspicions of doctors are misplaced. However, nearly a third (32.8 per cent) of respondents had alleviated symptoms with possible life shortening effects (the so-called doctrine of double effect, where doctors knowingly prescribe pain-relief drugs which have the side effect of hastening death), and a similar proportion (30.3 per cent) had made decisions not to treat end stage conditions, knowing that this would hasten an inevitable death. Doctors did not think that a new law would make much difference to their palliative care philosophy.

## Safeguards in assisted suicide legislation

If assisted suicide were to be legalised, appropriate safeguards would be necessary to protect vulnerable people and prevent abuse. These would govern eligibility for assistance to die, the decision making process around death, and the broader cultural and social context within which assisted suicide was made available.

First, disabled people and terminally ill people need to have access to independent living and the full range of support services. Choices about death should not be made because life has been made unbearable through lack of choices and control. Moreover, palliative care is not currently available in many parts of the country. Palliative medicine can reduce pain and suffering at the end of life: assisted suicide is not an alternative to palliative care, but an addition to it. Some countries where assisted suicide is permitted have not made a commitment to palliative care, which makes it more likely for dying people to choose to end their lives prematurely, from fear of preventable pain and suffering. The broader cultural context is also important, because assisted suicide should not be promoted via negative images of disability and dying. Some of the advocacy around assisted suicide has stigmatised dependency and disability, and encouraged people to think that disability is a fate worse than death. Assisted suicide should be viewed as a last resort for a minority of people with terminal illness, not the expected and preferred option when faced with difficulty and disability.

Second, promoting autonomy should be balanced with protection, even if this verges on paternalism. Questions of definition need close attention in developing regulation of assisted suicide. The distinction between 'people with terminal illness' and 'terminally ill people' is very important, and not easy to specify. It is an important principle that the qualification for assisted suicide is the end stage of incurable disease accompanied by unbearable suffering. Simply being a disabled person is not a reason to be permitted assisted suicide. To broaden the eligible class too widely might be to put disabled people at risk in the way that critics fear.

Moreover, it is normal to fear disability and death, and it is often traumatic to incur or be diagnosed with incurable impairment or terminal illness. For example, Disability Awareness in Action quote Dr Ian Basnett, a quadriplegic, as saying of the period after the accident which left him quadriplegic, 'I was ventilator dependent for a while and at times said to people "I wish I was dead!" I am now extraordinarily glad no one acted on that and assisted suicide was not legal' (Hurst, n.d.). Experience shows that the initial anger and distress at diagnosis often gives way to a more balanced and accepting attitude over time. Therefore, people who have recently developed or been diagnosed with impairment or terminal illness should be prevented from exercising the choice of assisted suicide. There should be a short-term infringement of autonomy for newly disabled people, until they come to terms with their situation. Understanding the complex fears and yearnings of those who desire euthanasia is important (Wood Mak and Elwyn, 2005).

Moreover, even people in the eligible category may not always be able to make a rational decision to request death. For example, depression and other mental illness could cloud judgement and may prevent a person with terminal illness making a competent decision to request death. The right to request assisted suicide should depend on the mental competence of the person with terminal illness. Disabled people may become depressed at pain and restriction, and express desire to die. For example, Alison Davis (2004) discusses a phase in her life when this was the case for her. She fears that had it been legal, she would have requested assistance and suggests that most requests for death stem from depression.

Any request for assisted suicide should be subject to calm and careful scrutiny from both medical and legal professionals. Once a request has been made and approved, there should be a 'cooling-off period' for the person to consider their situation, at the end of which they should have to confirm once more that they understand the consequences of their decision and want to go ahead with assisted suicide.

Assisted suicide should only ever be available in very restricted circumstances: the end stage of terminal, incurable illness, when suffering becomes unbearable. Legalisation and regulation should be carefully framed, to ensure that the 'slippery slope' which opponents fear cannot occur.

## Conclusion

Listening to the voices of disabled people and those directly affected is an important principle in bioethics. It is dangerous for non-disabled people to project their own fears and misconceptions as to what it might be like to be impaired: as Iris Marion Young (1997) has argued, it is not easy to put yourself in another person's shoes and imagine what their quality of life is like. It is equally important to analyse and challenge the voices of disabled people. For example, much of the vocal opposition to assisted suicide does not engage closely with arguments about assisted suicide in the particular situation of end stage terminal illness, which is the only situation where Lord Joffe – or myself in this chapter – have advocated assisted suicide. The majority of people eligible for this measure would be people suffering from cancer. The vast majority of disabled people would not be covered by the measure. For example, it would not permit people like Elizabeth Bouvia, who was disabled but not terminally ill, to have assistance to end their lives. For me, support for assisted suicide in end stage terminal illness is not the same as support for voluntary euthanasia for disabled people, which I oppose for many of the reasons given by other disability rights commentators. There is an important difference between encouraging disabled people to die, and enabling dying people to die better.

Alison Davis (2004) argues that the legalisation of assisted suicide would lead to medical science being less concerned to cure illness or alleviate pain: rather than trying to do something about end of life situations and prolong life, doctors would prefer to sit by and allow people to die. This seems to be implausible. The whole of modern medicine is directed at trying to cure illness and keep people alive. The problem for many patients at the end of life is not so much that their doctors are eager for them to die, but that doctors find it very difficult to stop trying to help, to enable them to die naturally and have a good death. The reality is that people have to die of something.

Moroever, the vocal opposition of many disability rights groups and commentators to assisted suicide is not the whole picture. Many people who are in end of life situations request and desire assistance to achieve a good death. Surveys have found that the majority of disabled people and of the general population are in favour of assisted suicide. Even some disabled people's organisations – for example, Jerome Bickenbach (1998) cites the Coalition of Provincial Organisations of the Handicapped in Canada – have supported assisted suicide.

Allowing people to kill themselves with medical assistance would be a major step. Fears about the vulnerability of disabled and terminally ill people are not without foundation, even though they appear to me to be over-exaggerated. The question becomes an empirical one: does the the benefit to those who may choose to use assisted suicide, or who may be comforted by its availability, outweigh the threat to other people who may theoretically be pressurised into requesting the measure? Evidence from jurisdictions where assisted suicide is permitted – the Netherlands and Oregon – is not conclusive. However, in both countries, the vast majority of dying people do not opt for assisted suicide. Nor is there clear evidence of abuse of the law. After 30 years of assisted suicide in the Netherlands, there has not been an erosion of moral constraints nor extension to a wider class of disabled people. Since the Oregon Death with Dignity Act was enacted in 1997, fewer than 200 individuals have died as a result of lethal drugs prescribed by their physician (Miller *et al.*, 2004).

It is tempting to interpret some of the disability rights community's opposition to assisted suicide as arising from the dominance of social model perspectives. For those who claim that disability has nothing to do with impairment, or that disability should not be medicalised, it is simply inappropriate to talk in terms of disease, suffering and death, because the solution to the disability problem is removal of social barriers, independent living, social inclusion and respect, not attention to impairment. The power of social model approaches may have made it harder for the disability rights community to engage with debates about illness, impairment and end of life. Perhaps social model ideology enables some to disengage from troubling questions about bodies and mortality.

Whether or not this is true, it seems to me that disability rights-based objections to disabled people's exercise of autonomy at the end of life are procedural, not substantial. Given that the disability movement support disabled people to make choices in every other area of their lives, it seems inconsistent that disabled people should not be able to take control over the manner of their death. I believe that well-informed, well-supported, competent adults in end stage terminal illness should be able to exercise this choice. With suitable safeguards and regulation, I support the introduction of assisted suicide legislation.

# Part III

# The social relations of disability

# Chapter 9

# Care, support and assistance

## The complexity of care

Giving and receiving care is a biological imperative for human beings. Throughout the thousands of years of human existence, the fact that the period of youthful dependency lasts between ten and twenty years has necessitated care. For most societies, the corresponding dependency at the end of life has also generated complex social and cultural arrangements and obligations. Giving and receiving care is something which no individual can escape from at some points in the life cycle. This leads Abram de Swaan to argue that human beings are by nature interdependent: each depends on someone else, and in turn is needed by others. He exalts this practical necessity of mutuality into an issue of existential purpose and value – 'That is what conveys to people their significance for their fellow human beings and that is where they find the fulfilment of their existence' (de Swaan, 1990, 21).

However, the prevailing tradition of Western thought, based on notions of individual agency and centred on the public arena, neglects to explore or include the realities of care, dependency and interdependency within arguments about morality or politics. Instead, the assumption of a hypothetical being – usually male, unencumbered, physically and cognitively intact – enables the elaboration of patterns of rights and liberties which may bear little relation to the realities of life for the majority of citizens (just as Athenian democracy conveniently ignored slavery).

In this chapter, I weave a path through the complex forest of literature on care and dependency. I claim that some dominant voices in disability studies have failed to embrace the challenge of care, regarding it as an aspect of social oppression which can be eliminated, and replaced by the concept of independent living which can liberate all disabled people. Thus, for example, Michael Oliver suggests that dependency is not the inevitable consequence of impairment, but is created by the social, economic and political system in which disabled people live (Oliver, 1993). I agree with Oliver and others from the disability rights tradition that it is vital to situate particular care arrangements within the broader social and political context. I also agree that care has often been the site of oppression and disempowerment.

I would join with the disability rights movement in demanding systems of care and support which maximise independence and choice, and minimise abuse, neglect and paternalism. Yet I am sceptical as to whether the independent living model can achieve all that its advocates hope for. Further, I believe not only that dependency is inextricable from human existence, but also that many disabled people have needs which will inevitably generate forms of ongoing dependency which exceed typical time-limited dependencies.

Understanding that care and support relationships are complex, just as the people who receive care are diverse, may seem obvious, but the implications of this sometimes seem to be neglected within disability studies literature. The independent living movement was largely developed by adults with physical impairments, who wanted greater choice in their living arrangements, as well as access to mainstream employment and leisure opportunities (Williams, 1983). The help they required was usually with self-care, domestic tasks, and mobility. Yet this constituency is only one of many who each require different forms of care, help and assistance. The following list illustrates some of the range of those who may need to rely on some form of support:

- babies, children and young people;
- people with temporary illnesses or impairments;
- people with static permanent impairments;
- people with chronic or degenerative illnesses and impairments;
- people with terminal illnesses;
- people with mild to moderate learning difficulties;
- people with profound learning difficulties;
- people with mental health problems;
- people who are elderly and frail;
- people who are elderly and demented.

Of course, it is quite possible for people to be in multiple categories, or to move between categories. And although 'physically and cognitively intact adults' are not listed, they too require support and assistance in different ways, in particular when they become carers or helpers for people in one of these categories. It will be noted that the traditional independent living constituency is primarily drawn from the third and fourth of the ten categories.

As well as the range of people or life cycle points where support is needed, the help given may take hundreds of different forms, ranging from medical interventions, to self-care tasks, to domestic chores and driving, to advice, advocacy and emotional support, to protection. A third dimension of complexity is the relationships by which different forms of care are delivered to these different groups of people. For example, family members, friends, volunteers, statutory workers and paid assistants may be involved. And even within paid care, the level of professionalism varies – for example, between care assistants, nurses, social workers and doctors. Celia Davis (1998) makes useful distinctions between 'care giving', 'care work' and 'professional care', trying to extricate what care involves, and the role of the person who delivers it.

Of course, it is not just the disability movement which has selectively defined care. Confusions and difficulties have frequently arisen when accounts or relations of care are inadequate for the complexities of care. For example, Reynolds and Walmsley (1998: 66) argue that the dominant ideology of care relates to children, while the usual blueprint for services such as homecare is older people. This causes problems for disabled people, people with learning difficulties, and people with mental health problems who also use services (see also Lee-Treweek, 1996). Another example has been the drive of the carers' movement to define care narrowly in terms of unpaid voluntary care. Meanwhile, the disability movement has disowned the concept of care entirely (Wood, 1991). It is clear that ideas about care, definitions of care, and even terminology like 'care' itself, are inherently political. The care debate takes place within a society in which individuality and freedom are ever more strongly prioritised. Privacy and choice have become important values, and collectivism and interdependence seem to be out of fashion. It may be no coincidence that the disability movement's stress on independence and autonomy has coincided with the resurgence of the free market and of privatisation.

This chapter presents four moments in the debate on care and support. Each of these is a simplified sketch, intended to illustrate the unfolding of an argument over time and between perspectives. The first moment, summarised very briefly, is the traditional approach to care; the second is the disability rights critique of care; the third is the alternative account from the feminist ethic of care perspective. Each of those moments is presented as an antinomy, meaning the expression of a conflict or contradiction or paradox. The interests which collide are broadly those of carers, usually women, and those of people who need intimate help. The fourth moment represents my own attempt to reflect on the complexity of the social relations of care.

Ann Brechin suggests that there is a consensus that the aim of care should be 'promoting autonomy in the context of supported living' (Brechin, 1998: 175). This useful formulation has the advantage of being sufficiently vague to secure agreement from many stakeholders in the debate, but in this chapter I want to problematise it by suggesting that care and living arrangements are about more than autonomy and independence. Preferences around care and support also reflect competing ideas of what a good life may involve. While traditional institutions and suffocating paternalism should certainly be repudiated, there is also potential for harm within arrangements based on autonomy and individualism.

## Traditional care and its problems

Consequent to the industrial revolution, and developing ideas about otherness and difference, a whole class of individuals were excluded from productive labour, as simultaneously the family and the community became hollowed out by the demands of the capitalist economy. As a consequence, people with learning difficulties, physical impairments, and mental illness often became institutionalised, because there was no longer a family or a community network by which they could be maintained and supported in mainstream society. By the 1960s and 1970s, there was an emerging critique of institutional care, from a variety of perspectives. For example, there was a challenge to the practice of segregation, represented by the normalisation movement and by the disabled people's movement. There were a series of scandals about abuse and neglect in particular institutions. There were also concerns about the cost of maintaining large-scale establishments. During the 1980s these concerns, critiques and aspirations resulted in the movement towards community care. The National Health Service and Community Care Act 1990 represented the Conservative government's drive to promote care within the community, to close down institutions, to marketise welfare, and ultimately to reduce expenditure.

Alongside and against this tendency developed an important feminist critique of the ways in which care in the community meant care predominantly by women. Authors such as Dalley (1988), Finch (1984) and Ungerson (1987) challenged the assumption that caring was women's work, and the suffocation of women's freedom and aspiration which this represented. For them, the solution was a continuation of collective provision. Hilary Graham (1983) suggested that because women were the majority of carers, female identity was shaped by their involvement in caring, both in terms of labour, but also in terms of being people who cared for others emotionally. Meanwhile, a growing carers movement demanded respect and support for carers in the political arena, through the articulation of carers' rights. The problem with this debate was that the rights of disabled people, older people and others who received care were neglected. Implicitly or explicitly, these discourses on caring conceptualised cared-for people as a burden. Obscured was the fact that it was not just carers who were mainly women, but also that disabled people and older people were disproportionately likely to be female. It was not just women, but also disabled people who were being constructed through ideas about care (Morris, 1991).

## Independent living and its limitations

In earlier work (Shakespeare, 2000), I have suggested that traditional models of care could be conceptualised in terms of a colonial relationship (Memmi, 1990). The lives of disabled and older people are colonised by service providers. Broader structural relations – the failure of society to support and include vulnerable people – are obscured by focusing on the inadequacies of the individual. There is a tendency to view those who receive care as burdens, and to infantilise them. The colonising process comprises the way in which recipients of services are described, the way in which service users' voices are often ignored, and the way that the issue is constructed as a social problem.

Since the 1970s, a liberation movement has been challenging the colonisation of disability. The demand for a different approach to personal support has been central to the disabled people's movement. Civil rights and independent living have been the two key elements of the disability agenda. First, disabled people fought to escape from residential institutions. Second, disabled people fought to escape from care, and to establish forms of support which were more empowering. In the words of Richard Wood, then director of the British Council of Organisations of Disabled People, 'Let us state what disabled people do want by stating first what we don't want. WE DON'T WANT CARE!' (Wood, 1991: 201).

Jenny Morris has been at the forefront of conceptualising independent living. As a disabled feminist, she developed a critique of the feminist literature on caring in her 1991 book *Pride Against Prejudice*. In *Independent Lives*, she unpicked some of the ideas which independent living has reacted against, particularly the assumption that disabled people are inevitably dependent and helpless (Morris, 1993a). For Morris and other disabled writers, the vital distinction was between physical dependency – not being able to do particular tasks – and social dependency. The goal was not to learn skills and abilities, but to gain independence through being able to control how tasks are performed; 'The point is that independent people have control over their lives, not that they perform every task themselves' (Brisenden, 1989: 9). Previously, independent living skills had been about learning how to perform chores such as dressing and feeding. From a disability rights perspective, the aim became autonomy, not self-sufficiency.

Independent living, then, was based on living in an accessible home and the availability of accessible environments and services and information. The focus changed from the individual and their abnormalities and limitations, to the service environment, and how it could empower and facilitate. A vital element in the panoply of independent or integrated living services was personal assistance. Rather than relying on family, volunteers or carers provided by a local authority or voluntary organisation, disabled people demanded direct payments so that they could employ their own helpers.

The concept of the personal assistant represented a rejection of the care tradition in favour of a depersonalised model of help. Rather than relying on externally provided services, the individual was able to take control of their own lives, by dictating who provided help, and how it would be provided. The model assumed that care could be disaggregated into practical tasks, which were necessary, and emotional content, which was rejected. It also depended on the disabled person having the capacity and willingness to become an employer, managing the work of another person – often a team of other people. According to research by Vernon and Qureshi, the attitudes of the personal assistants are crucial:

> Respect, dignity, being treated equally, trust and reliability were all identified as critical factors in how service users felt about the service they received. At their best, relationships with staff maximised choice and control, reinforced self-esteem and dignity, and made users feel genuinely valued and care for; at their worst, they could enforce dependency and passivity, erode self-esteem and be intrusive.
>
> (Vernon and Qureshi, 2000: 272)

Conceptually, it is clear why direct payments/personal assistance offers huge benefits in terms of control and flexibility for disabled people. Disabled people have been able to employ staff who are compatible – in terms of gender, ethnicity and sexuality – and compliant with their own wishes. Empirically, the response from personal assistance users has consistently been very positive (Spandler, 2004). Financially, research has shown that direct payments schemes can be cost effective. Users have a strong incentive to use payments efficiently, and as employers they are responsible for administration and management (Zarb and Nadash, 1995). However, there are some important criticisms of this approach to providing care which should be advanced.

First, to what extent might the direct payments model replace traditional forms of care? Initially, there were considerable obstacles to the take-up of direct payments outside the narrow group of disability rights activists among whom the model was pioneered. Many local authorities were lukewarm at best, resistant at worst, to offering the option to disabled people (Pearson, 2004). An important factor in take-up is the existence of support services which can promote independent living, offer training, and facilitate disabled people to become employers of assistants. Support schemes have not been available in many parts of the country. However, since the Direct Payments Act, and with more support and promotion of the direct payments model, there has been a rapid increase in the number of disabled people receiving direct payments. For example, between 2002–03 and 2003–04 there was an 80 per cent increase in the number of adults receiving direct payments. However, the direct payments model remains a minority experience (Riddell et al., 2005). In 2003–04, while 96,700 of 18- to 64-year-olds received home care, only 11,300 received direct payments. Meanwhile, 67,300 disabled people aged 18–64 still received residential or nursing care (Department of Health Community Care Statistics 2003–04).

Despite the fact that the direct payments model seems desirable to many users, it may not be chosen by all disabled people. For example, some might prefer to receive support from a family member. Others may not want the stress of recruiting and managing staff or negotiating working relationships (Carmichael and Brown, 2002; Scourfield, 2005). People who are isolated, socially or geographically, may have difficulties recruiting suitable non-family assistants. At the moment, low take-up of direct payments is largely a matter of access, opportunity and familiarity. As these problems are overcome, a clearer distinction may develop between those who prefer to employ personal assistants, and those who prefer to continue with care provided in the traditional way. Nobody currently knows what proportion will opt for each solution.

Related to the question of reach is the issue of whether the direct payments model is equally appropriate for other groups who receive care. Take-up among people with learning difficulties (Askheim, 2003), people with mental health problems (Ridley and Jones, 2003), and older people (Payne et al., 1998) has been very slow. Again, this might either reflect users' unfamiliarity with the personal assistance concept, or it may suggest that the model needs to be adapted for different users, or it may even suggest that there are intrinsic drawbacks which make personal assistance less suitable for some people's needs.

For example, people with learning difficulties require different forms of assistance from people with physical impairments. Reynolds and Walmsley report on the type of support that is often provided by family members:

> The type of care offered by relatives of people with learning difficulties or mental health problems is usually quite diffuse, involving being available and responsible when they are needed, offering company, emotional support and often fighting for services.
>
> (Reynolds and Walmsley, 1998: 68)

While physically impaired people require basic tasks to be performed by personal assistants, people with cognitive impairments may be looking for advocacy, advice and emotional support. This erodes the separation of emotional from physical activities which has been implicit in the independent living model (Lynch and McLaughlin, 1995). Reynolds and Walmsley suggest:

> It would be challenging for people with learning disabilities or with mental health problems to separate out from the context of their close personal relationships, which may well involve considerable interdependency, those aspects of their care which can be seen as a commodity to be purchased.
>
> (Reynolds and Walmsley, 1998: 78)

There is also a class of people with profound learning difficulties who are never going to benefit from the flexible and individualised support that personal assistance offers (Vehmas, 2006). Those who are unable to exercise any but the most basic choices may not experience any difference between alternative forms of care: residential care, family care or independent living may be interchangeable, assuming that there is no abuse, and that needs are met. Discussing her very impaired daughter Sesha, Eva Feder Kittay writes,

> Independent living is a subsidiary goal to living as full and as rich a life as one's capacities permit. I believe that a focus on independence, and perhaps even on the goal of inclusion when inclusion is understood as the incorporation of the disabled into the 'normal' life of the community, yields too much to a conception of the citizen as 'independent and fully functioning'.
>
> (Kittay, 1999: 172)

For Sesha and many others lifelong dependency is inevitable, and the task becomes to try and provide stimulation and enjoyment, not to maximise independence.

These critiques are based on the relevance and acceptability of the model to potential users. Another class of problems arises when the situation of personal assistants themselves is considered (Scourfield, 2005). There has been a lack of research with people who give help within personal assistance relationships about their own experiences and values. Some tentative findings suggest that workers also value the flexibility and changed relationship with service users (Glendinning *et al.*, 2000). However, others have feared that the individualised relationship between employer and worker represents a threat to staff. Workers are less likely to be unionised than traditional local authority employees, and may be vulnerable to exploitation, for example through low pay and anti-social hours. Some disabled people have written of their preference for employing unskilled staff, because they can be trained by the user to meet their needs appropriately, rather than imposing their own ideas of what is best. Yet this might also make the worker vulnerable to harm – for example, through lifting or carrying in ways which cause back problems (Spandler, 2004: 191).

Even where the worker is safe and has good pay, terms and conditions, this does not necessarily mean that the personal assistance model is without problems. Other issues include difficulties in recruitment, potential confusion in roles, unreasonable expectations, quick turnover of staff and problems of confidentiality if personal assistants talk to each other, or the same worker is employed by different disabled people. These problems sound not dissimilar to the 'servant problem' which troubled the middle class in the mid twentieth century. Some authors have argued that the individualised relationship is a threat to socialised welfare, and risks a return to the pre-war era of the servant class (Graham, 1991; Williams, 2001). Perception of direct payments as a form of privatisation or marketisation by left-wing local authorities – and trades unions – may be an obstacle to promotion of the personal assistance model (Carpenter, 1994; Pearson, 2000).

This highlights an underlying tension in the employer/employee personal assistance relationship. The separation of practical from emotional tasks seems central to a model which is intended to replace care. Yet how desirable is it for either worker or employer to have a relationship which is devoid of attachment and care? I have witnessed a disabled person treating his personal assistants in a very formal and distant way: the worker sits somewhere else until called, is excluded from conversation, and is treated like the traditional servant. At the other extreme, I have witnessed a disabled person treating her personal assistant like a paid friend and confidante, more like a traditional 'lady's companion' than an employee. Each of these extremes seems problematic for the personal assistance model: the former, because it appears to replicate hierarchical servant relationships, the latter because it erodes the separation of practical and emotional roles on which independent living is based.

Figure 9.1 attempts to map the helper/helped relationship in a more nuanced way. One axis represents the level of control which the user has over the relationship. The other axis represents the extent to which the helper is distant and professional, at one extreme, and close and friendly, at the other. The personal assistance relationship could be largely formal, where the personal assistant is a helper, who responds to the wishes of the disabled person, but is kept distant. Or it could be more informal, where the personal assistant is as much a social

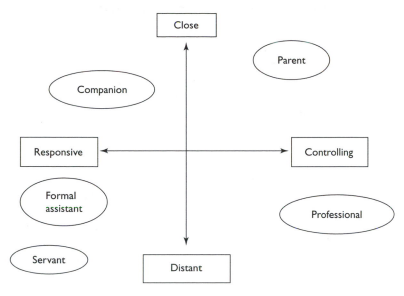

*Figure 9.1* The helper/helped relationship.

companion as a practical assistant. Looking at other helping relationships, a medical professional might be distant and formal, while respectful of the autonomy of the patient. A parent might be close and informal, but also potentially domineering and undermining of the disabled person's wishes. This approach to mapping the dynamics of the helping encounter suggests that a straightforward separation between tasks and affect is not necessary to a personal assistance relationship. Research from Japan confirms the multi-faceted relationships between disabled people and their assistants, where the latter were variously characterised as instruments, employees, companions and social assets (Yamaki and Yamazaki, 2004). Swedish research highlights the ambivalence and complications that can arise when young people have personal assistants, where power was often unequal and the relationship not mutual (Skär and Tam, 2001)

In recent years there has been an explosion of research and analysis of direct payments and personal assistance: this highlights the dramatic challenge which this model poses to traditional care, and the real benefits which it brings to disabled people (Stainton and Boyce, 2004). But these studies also document the variations (Askheim, 2005), barriers (Morris, 2004) and challenges (Maglajlic *et al.*, 2000; Carmichael and Brown, 2002; Scourfield, 2005) in this field. This evidence complicates the straightforward commitment of the disability movement to a simple model of personal independent living, showing that as provision expands, and as more groups are offered support, the picture becomes more complex and contested.

## The feminist ethic of care and its practicalities

Two alternative theoretical models for understanding and reforming care are currently available. One is based on the independent living principles which have been developed by the disabled people's movement. The second is the feminist ethic of care. Both share some criticisms of actually existing care, but provide significantly different strategies for developing new approaches. Disabled writers promote the civil rights of disabled people, and suggest that independence can be achieved via personal assistance schemes. Feminist writers favour replacing the discourse of rights with the discourse of care, and deconstructing the notion of independence itself. Yet engagement between the two perspectives has been minimal (Shakespeare, 2000; Watson *et al.*, 2004; Hughes *et al.*, 2005), despite the opportunities such partnership might offer for a more holistic programme of reform.

The feminist ethic of care originated partly in the work of psychologist Carol Gilligan, and particularly from her 1983 study *In a Different Voice*, which criticised the traditional models of moral development advanced by psychologists such as Lawrence Kohlberg. He argued that people advance through stages towards a moral competence which is based on abstract notions such as justice and equality. Yet Gilligan and others have suggested that Kohlberg privileged one particular way of looking at the world, and creating a hierarchy of moral competence which does not reflect the experience of women, for example. In contrast, feminists have suggested that women have alternative responses to moral problems, which are not inferior to those of men, but different.

Jean Tronto (1993) summarises three major distinctions between what has been called the 'ethic of rights', and the feminist 'ethic of care'. The ethic of care is based on relationships and responsibilities, while the ethic of rights is based on rights and rules. The former emerges from concrete circumstances, rather than formal and abstract situations. Finally, the ethic of care depends on activity, while the ethic of rights depends on principles. Drawing on these differences, feminist philosophers have argued that public discourse needs to draw on the neglected ethic of care, as a balance to the dominant ethic of rights, and they have elaborated the implications of this approach for welfare. For example, Eva Feder Kittay criticises the liberal contractarian framework developed by the philosopher John Rawls (1972). His approach cannot adequately include those who are dependent, and those who attend to their needs. She suggests, 'Once we stop ignoring dependency, then we are obligated to think of how dependency needs are met in a manner that is equitable to all' (Kittay, 1999: 90). Rawls' central idea of justice as fairness fails to meet these dependency concerns, and Kittay argues that his famous two principles need to be supplemented with a third, covering social responsibility for care.

From a disability studies perspective, one could develop some critiques of this approach. For example, there is a tendency in some of this literature to idealise the caring role, and to develop an almost essentialist idea of women as carers. Yet users of care services may well have reason to reject this for reasons highlighted earlier: they may feel taken over, spoken for, undermined, disempowered or even neglected and abused by carers. This reality goes against the overly romantic approach to caring work exemplified in the traditional carer literature, or for that matter in the work of feminist philosophers such as Nel Noddings (1984), who rarely if ever consider the care-receiver or the downside of care.

Moreover, the literature on the feminist ethic of care perhaps fails to grasp a key problem. Within the public sphere, it may be important to challenge the ethic of rights, which is variously described as patriarchal in essence or in values (Larrabee, 1993) and which depends on abstract universals such as equality and justice and the liberal concept of the independent, autonomous agent. A feminist ethic, with more or less essential overtones, is offered as an alternative based on relationships and responsibilities. In the public domain, the stress on interrelationships and interdependencies seems welcome. Yet, in the private sphere where much caring takes place, the contribution of the feminist ethic of care would surely be resisted by those who come from a disability rights perspective, who might argue conversely that the fundamental need is for the application of the ethic of rights to the social relationship of care. So, for example, disabled people have promoted the slogan 'rights not charity': the basic demand is for disabled people to receive personal assistance as of right, not to be dependent on care or kindness. As Anita Silvers argues, 'far from vanquishing patriarchal systems, substituting the ethics of caring for the ethics of equality threatens an even more oppressive paternalism' (Silvers, 1995: 40).

However, more recent writers from the feminist ethic of care position move away from the opposition of care and rights, and also show more understanding of the problems of disempowerment. For example, Sevenhuijsen and others have criticised what she calls 'the shadow side of virtue' (Sevenhuijsen 1998: 12), meaning the conflict, aggression and ambivalence which is also sometimes present in caring:

> Even if care is to a certain extent generated by dependency and attentiveness, the concrete motives in social practices of care cannot always be derived from the urge to protect dependent people from vulnerability. Caring for others can also stem from less noble motives, such as the urge to meddle or to control others.
>
> (Sevenhuijsen, 1998: 20)

Marilyn Friedman (1993) argues that justice and caring are mutually compatible: close relationships create special vulnerability to harm and abuse, she argues, and justice is relevant to rectification in this case. In her work, and that of others (Tronto, 1993), there has been some progress towards dissolving the false dichotomy of care versus justice. Certainly, one would want to support the argument that care can bring benefits to democratic citizenship, as long as it was also accepted that justice and equality may bring benefits to caring relationships and the private sphere: this, after all, has been a central part of the feminist project. A feminist ethic approach draws attention to the way that:

> In developing a masculinist approach to care, the disabled people's movement seeks to promote autonomy for disabled people but eliminates emotion from the caring process by transforming it into a formal, contractual, exchange relationship.
>
> (Hughes *et al.*, 2005: 271)

Fiona Williams has been central to this endeavour to reconcile rights and care, and is one of the few non-disabled feminists who have engaged deeply with the disability critique of care. She argues that people should not be fixed in a role as either carer or cared-for, because we are all givers and receivers: 'Care is an activity that binds us all' (Williams, 2001: 487). Vulnerability is part of the human condition. For Williams, personal assistance has an important part to play in the mixed economy of care. Across the range of options, the important values should be accessibility, affordability, variety, choice, quality, flexibility, control.

Reconciling the disability rights and feminist ethic of care approaches represents the way forward for understanding and improving the social relations of care (Hughes *et al.*, 2005). Yet two problems remain for me. First, how genuine is the idea of interdependence and reciprocity which lies at the heart of the ethic? There is a major difference in degree between the interdependence of non-disabled people, and the forced dependence of some people with impairments. As Eva Feder Kittay says,

> While the image of a mutuality and interdependence among persons is an important one, life with Sesha underscores that there are moments when we are not 'inter' dependent. We are simply dependent and *cannot* reciprocate. Furthermore, while dependence is often socially constructed – *all* dependence is not.
>
> (Kittay, 1999: 180)

To say that everyone is vulnerable, and that everyone gives and receives care is a truism which can become trite. Certainly, across the life span, everyone starts as a baby and most people end as an older person with care needs. Yet this 'conventional dependency' is very different from the extensive dependency experienced by some disabled people.

Reciprocity is an important factor in social relationships. Adults help each other, and over the long term the assistance usually balances out. Equally, across the life span, the support a parent gives to a child is often reciprocated when the child in his turn supports his own children, while possibly simultaneously caring for his own parents. Similarly, in a complex society, everyone depends on others to provide services and help out, and in turn most people contribute to the common good by the work which they do. Older people are supported by society, but have previously made their productive contribution. The case of significant impairment – whether physical or mental – is different. For example, Abraham de Swaan (1990) points out that illness leads to imbalance. A person who needs help, but cannot help others to the same extent, enters a relationship of dependency. She cannot return the favour, and consequently becomes indebted and inevitably loses some status in the interaction. Anita Silvers argues, in opposition to feminist ethic approaches, that

> Institutionalized caring depersonalizes whoever is cared for by shifting the source of the care-giver's motivation from affectional, admirational or reverential regard for the particular recipient of care to diligent regard for the social role of care-giver.
>
> (Silvers, 1995: 43)

It seems to me that both the disability rights movement and the feminist ethic of care perspective attempt to gloss over the problems which this causes. Feminists have discussed interdependence and caring solidarity, ignoring the inevitable inequalities in giving and receiving help. Disability activists have focused on direct payments and personal assistance, implying that dependency is a product of social arrangements, rather than individual functioning. Disability studies authors sometimes adopt a relativism and contextual essentialism which denies that many impairments do generate forms of dependencies. Thus Silvers claims, 'A specific impairment need have no natural or necessary deleterious impact on a life. Indeed, what counts as an impairment is itself relative to what is imagined to be normal, the last being, of course, a famously procrustean concept' (Silvers, 1995: 47). Similarly Jenny Morris argues, 'Physical impairment – the functional limitations which restrict what people can do for themselves – does not in itself create dependency' (Morris, 1993a: 87).

Statements like these seem to ignore the variations in impairment experiences, and the reality that the majority of disabled people do not operate the personal assistance model, and many will never be able to do so. When personal assistance works, it seems to liberate. But even personal assistance users are vulnerable to times when their support package collapses – because the worker is ill, or delayed, or fails to perform their role for any other random reason. The personal assistance users may not be dependent on care, as in the past, but they are now dependent on a package of personal assistance, and when it occasionally fails, they may again experience dependency because their physical limitations mean that they cannot do certain tasks which the vast majority of 'conventionally dependent' adults could perform. So independent living does not abolish dependency. There may be more or less dependency – and different kinds of dependency – and even differently valued dependency – but there is always dependency.

The second problem I have with the feminist ethic is a practical one. The approach seems strong on ideas, but short on detail. What would it mean, in practical terms? How would patterns of support be reorganised along feminist ethic of care lines? Can the feminist ethic of care be operationalised? The advantage of the disability rights approach is that it offers a model of independent living which can make a practical difference for thousands of disabled people. Perhaps the value of the feminist ethic approach is as critique: it points to the danger in complete espousal of independence and rights as a goal. It seems likely that the independent living solution of direct payments and personal assistance will not solve all the problems. Even within independent living models, disabled people still often depend on goodwill and mutual aid (as do everyone). As Alastair Macintyre argues,

> Market relationships can only be sustained by being embedded in certain types of local nonmarket relationship, relationships of uncalculated giving and receiving, if they are to contribute to overall flourishing, rather than, as they so often in fact do, undermine and corrupt communal ties.
>
> (Macintyre, 1999: 117)

The danger comes when disabled people are denied access to independent living, when they have no choice and no alternative, and are reliant on unresponsive services or demeaning charity which renders them marginalised and dependent. Yet empowered disabled people will achieve a better quality of life in a community in which each recognises their responsibility to the other, rather than a world made up of competing and selfish individuals seeking to maximise their own advantage.

## Complications and conclusions

By exploring three moments in the development of care and support, I have tried to show some of the complexities of the care debate. My aim is not to debunk independent living and direct payments, but to suggest that the situation is more complex and the solution not as complete as has been assumed in some of the disability studies literature. I believe that it is necessary to incorporate some of the insights of the feminist ethic of care perspective alongside the philosophy of independent living. I also believe that it is important to maintain a pluralist approach to providing care and support.

In order to map some of this terrain, a simplified matrix may have value (see Table 9.1). Caring arrangements are complex and multi-dimensional, comprising factors such as the place where care is provided, the relationships between recipient and provider, and whether the support is continuous or intermittent (Peace, 1998). Not all options are available for any individual disabled person. For example, living completely independently is only suitable for a disabled person who does not require regular personal assistance; direct payments is only an option in an area where these arrangements are provided for a person with a particular impairment; family accommodation and support depends on the existence of a willing parent or sibling.

This matrix is simplified, because it does not take into account all services an independent householder might use – for example, meals on wheels. Each cell

Table 9.1 A matrix of caring arrangements.

| | Companionship | Choice of companion/helpers | Agency | Flexibility | Privacy | Management responsibility | Risk |
|---|---|---|---|---|---|---|---|
| Independent householder | Potential isolation | Total choice | Total control | Total flexibility | High privacy | Total responsibility | High |
| Direct payments | Potential isolation | Choice within limits | High control | Flexibility within limits | Potential intrusions | Total responsibility | Low to high |
| Homecare | Potential isolation | Theoretical choice | Dependence on services | External routine | Intrusions from carers | Low responsibility | Moderate |
| Supported accommodation | Companionship | Minimal choice | Considerable control | Flexible within limits | Some intrusions | Low responsibility | Moderate |
| Family | Companionship | No choice | Potential paternalism | Flexible within limits | Lack of privacy | Low responsibility | Low |
| Residential care | Companionship | No choice | High dependency | Imposed routine | Lack of privacy | No responsibility | Minimal |

could be questioned: for example, companionship in family and aggregate living is not chosen; risk of accident may be minimised in collective living, but risk of abuse may be increased. A two-dimensional grid cannot effectively represent a multi-dimensional phenomenon, which is my underlying point. But at a general level, the diagram does show the plurality of available models, and how each can be associated with benefits and weaknesses.

The matrix shows a conventional gradient of independence, ranging from the freedom of an independent householder, to the dependency of someone living in residential care. The disability rights community have favoured values of autonomy and normality: forms of living which approximate to the age appropriate average are preferred, in which individuals can exercise as much control as possible over their lives. However, the point of the grid is to show that the more restrictive forms of living do have some advantages – in particular social contact and low responsibility – and that the more independent forms of living also have potential drawbacks – for example, isolation, and vulnerability if anything goes wrong (such as if someone has a fall or other emergency). An individual's preferences will depend on what they value in life, and on the details of each of the situations which may be available to them – for example, their relationship with parent or sibling and their particular constellation of needs and vulnerabilities.

What is not apparent from the matrix is that the most autonomous form of living, that of an independent householder – which resembles most closely that of the average, non-disabled member of society – is not free of dependencies or disadvantages. For example, so-called independent citizens depend on many different types of services – from refuse collection to housing maintenance to public transport to home delivery groceries and pizza – in order to survive in a busy, dangerous and complex world. The illusion of choice and control breaks down if the babysitter does not arrive, or if the municipal services go on strike, or if other external contingencies destroy the carefully nurtured illusion of individual autonomy.

The matrix attempts to describe the plurality of care and support models, and it highlights the costs and benefits of each. This suggests a conceptual point: any solution to the dilemma of care should not be seen as an end in itself, but as a means to an end. For example, independent living is a means of enabling an individual to have control over their life. Residential care may be a means of enabling an individual to have security. Care is not a single and simple goal, but can be disaggregated into a range of different goals, or ends. Different ways of providing support are not just different means to the same end, but often represent different means to reach different ends. The desirability of these different ends may depend on the particular idea of the good life which an individual or their family adopts. For example, the different ends which different people value might include:

- control over one's own life;
- convenience and lack of responsibility;
- safety and security;

- companionship and intimacy;
- routine and familiarity.

There are also different agents involved. These include the disabled person themselves; the parents or family of the disabled person; the people who deliver care services; the authority who is responsible for funding and organising care. Each of these may have their own set of goals for the helping situation, which may conflict. For example, some parents of people with learning difficulties may look to a living arrangement to deliver safety and security, and fear any arrangement which seems to imperil those ends by prioritising freedom or flexibility.

Any particular living arrangement may involve a trade-off between different ends. Safety may be gained at the cost of flexibility or control; independence may be gained at the cost of isolation. If this approach is correct, it suggests that the complexity of living options is poorly served by a rhetoric in which the different forms of care are ranked in a straightforward hierarchy, with a direct payments system at the top, as the best and most empowering approach for the majority of disabled people.

However, it may be that independent living based on direct payments represents the best compromise between the different ends for the average disabled person. For example, it may be possible for many direct payments users to achieve levels of convenience, control, companionship, safety and routine which are perfectly acceptable to them. But even if this is the case, there will be many other disabled people who favour different arrangements, because they value other ends more than choice and control: see, for example, those people with learning difficulties who like living in Camphill communities such as Botton (Rawles, 2004).

In this chapter I have argued for a pluralist approach to care and support, recognising the diversity of disabled people's lives and preferences. Independent living has transformed the choices for thousands of disabled people, but it is not the only approach to solving the problem of meeting physical and other needs. If autonomy and choice are regarded as the only desirable ends, then personal assistance schemes will always come out on top. But other disabled people may value other goals.

Debate on care and support should be based on the recognition that people are different in their support needs, in their aspirations, and in their values. Different forms of care are needed that support individuals in appropriate ways, which enable them to flourish and achieve their projects. One size will not fit all – either the historic form of residential care, or the current ideal of independent living. Whatever form of care and support is adopted needs to be based on respect for both parties – those who deliver care and support and those who receive it. In most cases, an individual will not be fixed into only one role, because the majority of humanity both receives and gives care at different points of the life course and in different relationships. It is wrong to think in terms of opposed interests and separate groups. All support and care systems need to balance individualism and mutuality, as Selma Sevenhuijsen suggests:

> The feminist ethic of care points to forms of solidarity in which there is room for difference, and in which we find out what people in particular situations need in order for them to live with dignity. People must be able to count on solidarity, because vulnerability and dependency, as we know, are a part of human existence: we need each other's disinterested support at expected and unexpected moments.
>
> (Sevenhuijsen, 1998: 147)

Regardless of the formal arrangements, the safety of the person receiving care and support is vital. Services need to be reliable, free from abuse, and minimise the vulnerability of the user. Warmth, care and respect should always be an important part of a personal assistance relationship. Equally, autonomy, independence and flexibility should be fostered within more traditional caring relationships.

# Chapter 10

# Disability rights and the future of charity

## Introduction

One of the consistent themes in the British disability rights movement has been a vehement opposition to charities which claim to represent and support disabled people. Many of the early activists of the Union of Physically Impaired Against Segregation (UPIAS) had come from the Le Court Cheshire Home in Hampshire. UPIAS itself had arisen in opposition to more mainstream charities and pressure groups run by non-disabled people. Throughout the 1980s and 1990s, demonstrations against charity fundraising – for example, the 1992 Block Telethon direct action – were important political events in the development of a disability rights consciousness, bringing together disability activists, and challenging traditional responses to disability. Key slogans of this period, seen on banners, placards, t-shirts and in the protest songs of Johnny Crescendo and Ian Stanton were 'Rights not charity' and 'Piss on pity'.

Opposition to charities continues into the twenty-first century (Rickell, 2003; Burrows, 2003). For example, the Direct Action Network (DAN) has campaigned vociferously against the major charities. In 2002, a group of DAN activists disrupted a Leonard Cheshire Foundation charity ball in Manchester, blockading the doors and letting off stink bombs. In November 2003, DAN staged a three-day protest outside four major charities – Scope, RNID, RNIB and Mencap. One protestor was quoted as saying at a meeting with Mencap: 'We are at war with you, and we will make sure we do as much damage as possible to you because you're not on our side' (Burrows, 2003). The disability activist opposition to charity can sometimes appear almost obsessive, such as the subscriber to *Disability Arts in London* (summer 2004, issue 182) who withdrew from BCODP and *Disability Arts in London* mailings because they took advertisements from Scope.

There is a paradox here. The public perception of charities is very positive. Many members of the public are motivated to contribute money to support the work of voluntary organisations providing services at home and abroad. Millions of people in need – children, older people, disabled people, people in developing countries – have been supported as a result of charitable donation and distribution. Where the private sector often seems self-interested, and government appears unresponsive and inflexible, charitable organisations have a reputation for innovation and direct practical assistance. Yet the British disability community denounce charities and call for them to be closed down.

The word charity has several meanings, according to the *Concise Oxford Dictionary*. First, 'love of fellow men; kindness; affection; leniency'. Second, 'beneficience, liberality to those in need or distress, alms giving'. But this second definition also lists ' institution for helping those in need'. The frustration and anger of the disability rights community seems to be directed towards charities as institutions. The claim of those who adopt the social model is that a world free of oppression and barriers, in which disabled people had full civil rights, would be a world in which charity was no longer required.

This chapter will explore and evaluate the disability rights community's critique of charity, asking whether opposition to charitable organisations is still justified in the twenty-first century, and exploring whether beneficence would become unnecessary in a world based on civil rights and equality. In presenting the disability rights critique, I will focus on three dimensions.

1   The difficulty of what charity symbolises.
2   The issue of what charities do.
3   The practical problems of how charities go about their business.

In each of these areas, the disability rights critique continues to have validity. However, I will conclude by claiming that, despite these merits, the critique as a whole is outdated and self-defeating.

## Charity as symbolism

Religious and humanitarian impulses mandate generosity and support for those in need. Jesus told the parable of the Good Samaritan; charity is one of the five pillars of Islam; Buddha was inspired by the suffering of the old, the poor and the disabled. But charity has often been criticised as being an inadequate response to the problem of disadvantage, which fails to solve the underlying problem, and also creates a relationship of dependency. As the philosopher Raymond Gaita suggests, 'Good-hearted people find it intolerable that just treatment of the powerless should depend on the generosity – in the charity in the old-fashioned sense – of the powerful' (Gaita, 2002: 201).

Charity tends to individualise need. Any problem may become perceived in terms of an incapable person requiring assistance from a capable person. This obscures the underlying causes of need. Activists argue that disabled people have been forced to rely on charity because they have been excluded from employment and from participation in society. It is not that disabled people are incapable, it is that they experience oppression and barriers. Charity, then, is an inadequate and inappropriate solution. Instead, the answer is to remove barriers, provide better services and empower people to be independent.

When a particular group of people is strongly associated with charitable provision, the result is to demean that group. Those who receive charity are regarded as unable to help themselves. People with power or resources volunteer to help those without power or resources, but the consequence is to make the latter feel dependent and incapable of surviving independently. The charitable relationship is an unequal one. Jerome Bickenbach argues, 'Since a recipient of charity is the beneficiary of another's virtue, a virtue denied to the recipient, charity creates a morally asymmetric relationship' (Bickenbach, 1993: 197). Symbolically, the institutionalisation of altruism through the organisation of charity remains a model influencing the way help is delivered and understood in British society, 'a concept of social relations in which some people are active agents and others just passive recipients' (Williams, 1989: 42).

The association of disabled people and charity suggests that disabled people have no option but to rely on handouts. It suggests that non-disabled people are beneficent and that disabled people are needy. It leaves disabled people feeling dependent and incapable. This discourse structures the way that non-disabled people relate to disabled people, and the way that disabled people feel about themselves. Researching disability identity, Nick Watson (2003) found that many of his respondents described their unhappiness with charitable discourse: some had even experienced being thrown coins in the street.

In particular, charities working in the disability field have historically individualised disability, representing it in almost exclusively medical terms. Charities have played a major role in the idea of disability as an individual tragedy. Donors have been manipulated into sympathy and generosity by the idea of awful diseases ruining the lives of people – often children. The marketing and advertising campaigns of the major medical research charities were expertly dissected by David Hevey (1992), who explored how charities 'market' impairments just as businesses 'brand' their products. For example, the MS Society specialised in grim images of dependent and desexualised adults with 'torn out' spines or eyes, and used the strap line 'tears lives apart' and 'a hope in hell'. These representations established the need for, and value of, the charity, while promoting a negative view of the people with the disease, paradoxically undermining the goal of acceptance and inclusion for disabled beneficiaries of the organisation. Disability was located firmly in the body – as opposed to in social exclusion – and the aim was to evoke pity and sympathy, and hence charitable donations. For Hevey, charity advertising was 'the calling card of an inaccessible society'.

It is easy to be cynical about charitable fundraising activity. Huge billboards advertising particular campaigns dominate urban areas and make disabled people feel inadequate or tragic. Disability becomes an tragedy, not a political responsibility. Celebrities gain positive publicity or atone for their mistakes by high-profile support for good causes. Television fundraising events, such as ITV's Telethon or the BBC's Children in Need are entertaining, and enable everyone who participates, watches or donates to feel better about themselves. Yet, for the disability rights community, the cost of these responses to the disability challenge outweighs the benefit. Charity enables the public and the politicians to feel that the problems have been solved, and that there is nothing they need to worry about. Paul Longmore (1997) argues that giving to fundraising enables Americans to escape the mood of futility and fatalism, achieving revalidation through believing they can transcend the human condition. Charity reinforces the idea of disabled people as dependent: in the words of Barnes and Mercer (2003: 26), charity offers 'an enduring cultural message that helps perpetuate an image of helplessness and dependency'. As Robert Drake argues, 'Disabled people demand the opportunity to acquire resources through work, rather than to receive largesse through public subscription. Many are angered by their portrayal as objects of pity; an image damaging to their dignity and social standing' (Drake, 1996: 157).

## Charity as provider

A second area where the disability rights movement has been critical of charity relates to the types of services and activities which charities tend to provide, which could be seen as the antithesis of the values and strategies adopted by disabled people's organisations (Campbell and Oliver, 1996). Looking at the origins of disability charities highlights the disparity.

Some charities date back to the Victorian period, and were founded in order to support people with particular impairments: for example, the Royal National Institution for the Blind and the Royal National Institution for the Deaf. These charities aimed to support a particular impairment group who were in need, and developed homes, schools and sheltered workshops. At this time, the traditional support structures of family, church and community were being eroded by the rapid transition to an urban industrial capitalist economy. Moreover, there was greater awareness and concern about those who were socially excluded. In the absence of state support, philanthropists were motivated to provide segregated forms of provision.

Other charities have sprung up in the post-war period, often as responses to particular medical problems. For example, the National Spastics Society, forerunner of Scope, was founded in 1952 by a group of parents of people with cerebral palsy, in association with a social worker. In 1963 this merged with the British Council for the Welfare of Spastics to become The Spastics Society, which developed into a major provider of educational and residential services for people with cerebral palsy. Self-help groups have been formed to support individuals and families affected by many different medical conditions, providing information and advice, and sometimes advocating for better provision, but usually not becoming service providers. Typically, doctors and parents have worked together to initiate these groups. In the case of degenerative or life-threatening diseases, charities have been formed to raise funds for scientific research into the conditions: again, parents and medical scientists have often been the driving force.

From a disability movement perspective, these charitable responses are problematic because each organisation caters for people with a particular type of impairment.

Although there are some disability rights organisations which serve a single constituency – for example, the British Deaf Assocation – the tendency is to have cross-impairment groups which organise on a geographical basis, such as the Greater Manchester Coalition of Disabled People or the Greater London Association of Disabled People. From a social model perspective, organising according to impairment suggests that impairment is the dominant problem for disabled people, and ignores the shared experience of oppression which unites disabled people. The focus on medical research and treatment which is a feature of many charities further contravenes the social model claim that disability is a social creation, not an individual medical tragedy.

Many charities have historically offered services on a segregated basis, another point of concern for disabled people. For example, the Leonard Cheshire Foundation, Scope, RNID and RNIB have all provided residential care and special schools. The disability rights movement is committed to inclusive education and to independent living in the community. The Direct Action Network has explicitly identified residential provision as a main source of disagreement: the slogan 'Free our people', and the description of residential homes as 'plantations' implies that the disability charities are incarcerating or enslaving disabled people against their will (Campbell and Oliver, 1996: 131).

Finally, where the disability movement has campaigned for civil rights legislation and social change, historically disability charities have downplayed political activity. Legal restrictions prevent party political activity by charities, and tightly constrain the extent to which they can campaign to change the law. Disabled people's organisations have long believed that the solution to disabled people's problems is in new statutes, such as anti-discrimination or direct payments legislation. Only belatedly did the major charities join the Rights Now campaign to help achieve civil rights protection.

## Charity as organisation

The third element of the disability rights critique concerns the governance, ethos and profile of disability charities. Again, a series of contrasts are drawn between the charitable sector and the disability rights sector, the difference often being described as that between charities as 'organisations for' and disability groups as 'organisations of' (Oliver, 1990).

Historically, charities have been managed and staffed by non-disabled people. Often it has been 'the great and the good' who have served as patrons. In the case of post-war charities, doctors and parents have initiated and directed the work, and as charities have grown professional managers have taken over operations, often with no previous experience of disability. Many charities have failed to employ members of the populations they have served (Prasad, 2003). Not only have charities been run by non-disabled people, but they have also been unresponsive to the expressed views of disabled people. Robert Drake's research with Welsh disability charities in the 1990s found that only very limited consumer participation had been achieved. Often the involvement of users was compartmentalised, and kept away from the main decision making structures (Drake, 1996, 160): there had been no fundamental shift in the balance of power within these organisations. When Drake (1996) interviewed non-disabled people who ran charities in Wales, they tended to see it as natural that voluntary groups should be run by non-disabled people. Disabled people were seen as passive recipients, who were prevented by their physical or mental limitations from taking leadership roles.

Whereas the majority of charities are small self-help organisations, some disability charities have become very large indeed (Harris and Rochester, 2001). The huge disparity in government funding to organisations 'for' rather than organisations 'of' has been a traditional criticism in the disability studies literature (Oliver, 1990). Community care reforms in the early 1990s funnelled more funding towards disability charities, which took on contracts to provide services. Some organisations run by disabled people also managed to be funded under these changes, but generally there were fewer disability rights groups who had the skills and size to be able to benefit from the changes in welfare provision. The 'Big Five' organisations – Leonard Cheshire, RNID, RNIB, Scope and Mencap – are huge businesses, with turnovers in the region of £100 million. In order to attract suitable chief executives, they have offered salaries at a commensurate level, far beyond what the average disabled person earns. Few disabled people have had the experience or skills necessary to run these multi-million pound organisations, and therefore non-disabled chief executives have been the rule. Charity accounts, like those of similarly sized businesses and agencies, also reveal considerable spending on items such as public relations and administration. To disabled critics, all this implies that donations do not benefit supposed beneficiaries, but instead are diverted into salaries and overheads. It has been claimed that disability charities are self-serving, existing largely for the benefit of the staff who are employed in them. There are certainly a few charities of whom this is a just critique: they amass large financial reserves, while not benefitting their users to the extent that their resources might imply.

By contrast to the large disability charities, disabled people's organisations have historically been run largely by volunteers, have been poorly funded, and have a membership mainly or exclusively made up of disabled people. Disability rights groups have tended to be small organisations, fostering debate and information sharing and with close contact between membership and management. Struggling to survive and to promote a disability rights argument, activists have long resented the dominance of the traditional charities within the disability sector.

## Evaluating the critique

While it has certain merits, the disability rights critique of charities appears one-sided and exaggerated. It also fails to contextualise charities in the historical situation in which they emerged. For example, with hindsight, the creation of segregated living, educational and employment situations would now appear inappropriate and misguided. But at the time when charities were developing these services, this reflected contemporary thinking on the best ways to support disabled people. In the absence of segregated charitable provision, many disabled people would have been totally neglected. Until 1893, it was only voluntary charitable organisations which made any formal provision for disabled people (Topliss, 1979). Judging a previous historical era in terms of the standards and expectations of our own is not always appropriate or helpful.

Equally, the disability rights critique of the major charities has not evolved to take into account the changes that have occurred over recent years. Reviewing the history and literature of disability rights, the UK disabled people's movement gives the impression that it has a blanket opposition to charity, and that a firm political dichotomy has been established between organisations of (i.e. disability rights groups) and organisations for (i.e. charities). In the 1970s, when the disability movement was coalescing, the classic disability rights account of charity was largely accurate. Most charities reflected dominant ways of thinking about disability: that it was a medical issue, that non-disabled people had a religious and social obligation to support disabled people, that disabled people could not speak for themselves or look after their own affairs. Many of the key activists in the disability movement had lived in institutions run by charities, or attended segregated schools, and in a few cases even worked for charities. They had personal experience of being segregated and patronised and spoken for. Therefore their opposition to charities was founded on bitter experience, and was personal as well as ideological. Thirty years on, the voluntary sector has changed in many ways, and some of the disability rights challenges appear outdated and in need of updating.

It is important to note that the disability movement's public position has always concealed certain inconsistencies. In the early days of the British Council Of Organisations of Disabled People (BCODP), there were long discussions as to whether it should apply for charitable status. Today, it has charitable status, just like many other disabled people's organisations, for example the Greater London Association of Disabled People, the Derbyshire Centre for Inclusive Living, and the Council of Disabled People Warwickshire and Coventry. In the early days, the founders of BCODP wrote begging letters to major businesses asking for charitable donations (Campbell and Oliver, 1996: 79). Today, like many other disabled people's groups, BCODP is not shy of appealing for charitable donations: according to the 2003 annual report it has been the subject of a BBC Radio 4 charity appeal, and has received funding from Comic Relief, the National Lottery, Lloyds TSB Foundation, Joseph Rowntree Foundation and the City Parochial Foundation.

However, although the disability rights rhetoric is often stuck in the 1970s, the major disability charities have changed out of all recognition, partly due to wider political and social changes – such as community care policies which led to services being contracted out to the voluntary sector – but also as a result of the lobbying and protest of disabled people and their organisations. As Mike Oliver has said,

> My perception is that these organisations did not change because there were
> moles working from the inside, they changed because we became so powerful
> externally that they had no choice. They didn't want to look like what they are
> – which is nineteenth century remnants with no place in a modern welfare
> state.
>
> (Campbell and Oliver, 1996: 193)

Research with voluntary organisations in the disability field show that at least
superficial acceptance of social model thinking is now commonplace (Stalker
*et al.*, 1999: 14). Other signs of this change towards disability rights thinking
include the switch that several charitable trusts and foundations – including Charity
Projects (Comic Relief), National Lottery and Platinum Trust – made during the
1990s towards prioritising funding for disabled-led initiatives. As a consequence,
many disability rights organisations have benefited from financial support from
these sources, another fact which appears inconsistent with the blanket opposition
to charity.

In addition, the governance and values of major charities are changing. Many
disability charities are now formally majority controlled by disabled people. For
example, the Royal Association of Disability and Rehabilitation (RADAR), which
was once known as the Central Council for the Care of Cripples, now has a majority
of disabled people on its management committee, and a disabled chief executive.
A key example here is Scope, which changed its name from the Spastics Society
in 1994. For some years it has had a majority of disabled people on its governing
council. In 2003, it poached Andy Rickell, then the chief executive of BCODP, to
become a senior manager (Benjamin, 2004). In 2004, Scope launched both a high
profile civil rights campaign, Time To Get Equal, and a policy of reserving senior
management positions for disabled people, in an attempt to reach the target of
20 per cent of disabled staff by 2006 (it currently employs 3.4 per cent disabled
staff, but mainly in lower positions in the organisation). Scope is also committed
to ending segregated provision (Carvel, 2005): it has 500 people living in its
residential settings, and 300 children in its schools, half of whom receive some of
their education in inclusive settings, and the intention is to redirect these services
towards supporting inclusive education and independent living.

Third, there have been changes in charity advertising. The old formats, using
images of medical tragedy to prompt pity, are rarely seen. Organisations such as
Scope and Mencap now explicitly attack disability discrimination in their advertising, and Leonard Cheshire Foundation similarly uses the word 'enabled' to
connote its awareness of new disability discourse. Each of these organisations
promotes research and campaigning into discrimination and social exclusion.
Rather than giving credit for these improvements, disability activists continue to
be rejectionist and even to criticise the charities for adopting disability rights
rhetoric (Carr, 2000; Carvel, 2004).

Just as the traditional charities have changed, so have disability rights organisations. Some disability rights groups and other disabled-controlled self-help

groups have developed in size and skills. For example, community care policies have enabled centres for integrated living to become service providers, including running personal assistance schemes. This has led to increased funding, organisational growth, and the replacement of grass-roots activism and volunteering with more businesslike and professionalised approaches. As they grow, disabled-led service provision organisations come to resemble charities in their business methods, and run the same risks of losing touch with the grass-roots.

All this suggests that the traditional disability rights dichotomy between 'organisations for' and 'organisations of', which may have appeared useful in the 1980s, now fails to represent the complexity of organisations working with disabled people. The landscape of disability voluntary organisations is diverse in form and ethos, and cannot simply be divided into 'disability rights organisations' and 'charities'. Charities have become more like disability rights groups, and disability rights groups have become more like charities.

Adding to the complexity, there is now a new generation of user-led non-social model organisations (Goodley, 2003: 125). A typical hybrid is the Spinal Injuries Association (SIA), which was 30 years old in 2003 and is a registered charity. According to the 2003 Annual Report, it has grown to a turnover of £2,153,195. It employs 30 staff, more than half of them disabled people. The President, chair and trustees, and chief executive are all disabled people. It is a member of BCODP, and its annual report has a contribution from Mike Oliver, one of its founder members: Mike Oliver and Frances Hasler (1987) argued strongly for the SIA's self-help approach. Yet since 1984 SIA has had Princess Anne as its patron, and it relies on all the traditional means of fundraising: charity balls, lunches and sweepstakes, donations from charitable trusts and corporate sponsorship, even selling Christmas cards. Its aims are integration and participation, but alongside social and campaigning activities it also supports medical services and research.

Another important question is the extent to which the disability rights critique represents majority opinion among disabled people. In practice, disabled people have diverse views and desires. Charities have been criticised for being undemocratic and unrepresentative. Yet to my knowledge, there has never been a representative survey of disabled people's attitudes to charities, so it is impossible to know who best represents the views of Britain's ten-million odd disabled people or has their support. It is undoubtedly the case that many disabled people and their families benefit from the services provided by charities. For example, 25,000 people used Scope services in 2004, while 150,000 use RNIB. Often, it is disabled people themselves – or their families – who are promoting forms of segregated provision. People who have lived in residential institutions all their lives may not want to move into the community, or may feel unable to manage independently. Parents may campaign for special schools for their children, believing that their needs will not be met in the mainstream, or that they will be bullied.

Charities are not perfect institutions, and some of the smaller and more traditional charities are urgently in need of reform. However, the major disability charities who are the target of activist anger, probably do not deserve such attacks. Hostility towards charity is partly a legacy of early decades, and partly a function of the way that identity politics relies on having external enemies to bolster group coherence. A more rational approach would be more selective in its critique, and recognise the successes as well as the failures of the charitable sector. My analysis suggests that in many ways the disability rights critique of charity is now outdated: it was probably always simplistic.

## Living without charity

Many activists have called for an end to charity. In this section, I want to ask whether disabled people can survive without it. This is a question which could be asked in several different ways. First, should there be any voluntary organisations with charitable objects working with disabled people? Second, should the existing disability charities be closed down or handed over to disabled people? Third, does the charitable ethos itself still have a place in disability policy?

Without voluntary organisations, disabled people's needs could only be met by their own families, by the market, or by the state. Families and informal carers are already under extreme pressure, and disabled people have made it clear that they do not want to be dependent on relatives. Given the poverty of disabled people and consequent lack of purchasing power, it seems unfeasible for them to meet the needs for accomodation, support, counselling, transport and other services in the open market. Where the market has expanded – for example dominating provision of residential homes for older people – it is not clear that commercial providers offer better quality or more responsive services than either voluntary or statutory alternatives. Some countries, particularly the Nordic countries, have much more extensive state provision than the UK. However, this depends on much higher rates of taxation, which do not currently appear to be a practical political option in the UK. Moreover, state provision has a tendency to be monolithic, inflexible and unresponsive to individuals.

There have been claims that charitable assistance is only required due to the shortfall of mainstream provision or the failures of social organisation. For example, Robert Drake asks:

> Were disabled people to command incomes and resources through paid work, and were the social and physical environment suitably adapted so as to remove the obstacles that currently deny disabled people their citizenship, what kinds of duties would then remain for the statutory and voluntary services to perform?
>
> (Drake, 1996: 163)

This suggestion assumes that paid work is a realistic option for all disabled people: earlier in this book, I concurred with Paul Abberley (1996) in doubting that. For example, many people with profound learning difficulties or complex physical and sensory impairments may never be able to work. Similarly, the idea of a completely barrier-free world seems utopian. It is true that access to work and barrier removal might reduce considerably the number of disabled people who rely on support from the voluntary sector. The increasing independence and social participation of disabled people has already had this effect. But voluntary organisations still give very important support to disabled people and their families, and it is hard to conceive of a world where this would not continue to be the case.

Voluntary organisations have many advantages as providers of support and services to disabled people. Indeed, the entire disability rights movement is itself a part of the wider voluntary sector. At their best, voluntary organisations can be flexible and dynamic, and responsive to needs. They are often the source of innovation in services. See, for example, groups for rare or unsupported conditions such as Connect, the aphasia charity discussed in Swain *et al.* (2003: 92–97). Voluntary organisations can emerge from the communities they serve, and adopt the cultures and values of their clients – for example, organisations created by the gay community at the outset of the HIV/AIDS epidemic lead the way in respectful and responsive provision. Similarly, voluntary organisations from minority ethnic communities can overcome barriers and prejudices and understand particular cultural needs. At their best, charities can be moral leaders: they can speak out, they can set standards and spread ideas (Saxton, 1997).

It is also hard to imagine a world without medical research charities. Without independent fundraising by the charitable sector, medical research would be considerably limited. Government contributions to research are outweighed by those given by charities such as the Wellcome Trust, or by the major disability charities. In 2003, the 111 charities who are members of the Association of Medical Research Charities contributed over £660 million to fund research into both common and rare conditions. Some activists would argue that medical research was an inappropriate response to disability. Elsewhere in this book I have argued that many disabled people do not have the luxury of doing without medical research. For those with degenerative impairments such as cystic fibrosis or muscular dystrophy, medical research funded by disability charities offers hope of a future in which the conditions could be alleviated or cured.

The idea of abolishing the disability voluntary sector seems a brutal response to the problems of charity, and cannot be the goal of any but the most extreme of activists. However, many who would accept the need for some kind of disability voluntary sector – in other words, the continual existence of some form of disability charities – would nevertheless like to see the end of actually existing charities. For example, in 1996, the disability rights leader Jane Campbell argued:

> The help that these organisations have given to disabled people has been infinitesimal when compared with the hindrance they have caused and the damage they have inflicted. They have influenced disabled people to reject their bodies and minds, to regard their impairments as a tragedy which must be eradicated at any price, and to return to some mythical perception of undamaged normality. They have inflicted vast damage to disabled people's

self-worth. So, I would say that I would like to see an end to the impairment charities.

(Campbell and Oliver, 1996: 195)

I have argued above that this type of disability rights rhetoric regarding charity appears stuck in the past. It is not clear that organisations such as RNID, RNIB, Scope, Mencap and Leonard Cheshire now fit Campbell's description, even though her words may have been accurate thirty years ago. These organisations are changing, and should be supported to make further changes, in order to make them more responsive to disabled people and their families, and more relevant to the modern era. Current and continuing opposition appears like revenge against the abuses and failures of the past.

Some have argued that existing charities should be taken over by disabled people, or that funding should be switched to organisations controlled by disabled people. There are practical and conceptual reasons to question this suggestion. Looking at the experience of self-organised disability rights organisations suggests that they are not themselves immune from problems. While there are many well-run and professional disabled-led organisations, there are also many examples of failing organisations or failed projects. For example, there have been many incidents of bad employment practice in disabled people's organisations. There have been problems with racism, sexism and homophobia. Management committees of disabled people have sometimes lacked skills and professionalism. Poor selection procedures – or over-zealous commitment to employing only disabled people – have led to the appointment of disabled people who were incapable of performing effectively in their roles. Funding has been secured for initiatives – such as Disability Writes, a 1990s project to develop a national disability magazine – which have failed to deliver effectively.

These problems are not specific to disabled people's organisations: similar stories can be found in many other community organisations and campaigns. Equally, there are many professional and businesslike disabled-led organisations. It is also true that there are major constraints on the effectiveness of disabled people's organisations, which often lack proper funding for their work, and rely on volunteers. Disabled people themselves sometimes lack confidence, or education, or experience, as a result of wider patterns of disability discrimination. However, the reality of disability-led groups does suggest that the call by the Direct Action Network for charities to be handed over to disabled people would not be an automatic benefit. Given that the big charities have annual turnovers of up to £100 million, and that the largest disability movement organisations have turnovers of £2–£3 million, it could be inferred that the disability movement does not currently have the capacity to run such major operations.

Conceptually, there is a frequent assumption that disabled-led initiatives must be best. This does seem common sense. After all, disabled workers will be good role models for the disabled people with whom they work. Disabled managers will understand the realities of disabled people's lives better. Disabled workers will have the passion and commitment to make change happen. For example, it is often suggested that disabled people's organisations are best equipped to promote direct payments and independent living. However, it is not clear that this assumption must always be true. As I suggested above, some disabled-led organisations have been inefficient, incompetent and guilty of bad practices. It is quite possible to imagine an organisation staffed or run by non-disabled people which was committed to supporting disabled people and which performed more effectively. Particular organisations are a means to an end, not an end in themselves. While usually disabled people's organisations will be better (for example, at achieving high take-up of direct payments), sometimes the self-organised group may not be the best available option.

## Conclusion

Opposition to charity plays a powerful role in mobilising disability activists. Charitable organisations and their activities provide a convenient target for anger and frustration. Direct action builds a positive sense of identity, promoting a sense of disabled activists fighting non-disabled oppressors. Demonstrating against charity subverts and disconcerts public understanding of disability and the appropriate responses to it. Yet, in order to achieve and sustain this opposition, an outdated and one-sided picture of the role of charities has been created. Any changes which charities have made over the last three decades have had to be ignored. Charities are castigated if they ignore disability rights criticisms, but not rewarded if they then develop in appropriate directions.

While the disability rights movement has adopted the slogan of 'rights not charity', I argue that disability rights is not incompatible with charity. Removing barriers to participation and promoting the rights and independence of disabled people is the major priority, and charity is no substitute for this equalisation of relations between disabled and non-disabled people. The Jewish philosopher Maimonides favoured forms of charity in which there was anonymity of donor and recipient, because these prevented stigma and indebtedness. Yet the highest place on his 'golden ladder of charity' was reserved for interventions which removed the structural conditions which made people dependent on the generosity of others.

However, voluntary organisations and charitable relations will continue to be necessary, both on the road towards a more equal society, but also even after equality has been achieved. This is because disabled people and their families will continue to have complex needs, and voluntary organisations will often be the best way to support those needs. Charities need to continue to change: for example, research suggests that only about 50 per cent are innovative, and only 50 per cent have users on their governing bodies (Taylor, 1997). Charitable provision will need to be more responsive to the rights and dignity of disabled people and their families. It will have to be offered on the basis of partnership between disabled and non-disabled people: what Selma Sevenhuijsen (1998) has called 'caring solidarity'. Voluntary organisations, according to Robson *et al.* (1997: 17), are based on three values: caring for others (including philanthropy); mutual help (reciprocation between people in similar circumstances); empowerment and equality (solidarity to achieve change). While disabled people's organisations usually concentrate on the second and third value, and mainstream organisations often prioritise the first and second value, all three are relevant and important, and all three can provide a positive basis for improving the lives of disabled people.

The fundamental ethic underlying charity can only be positive, even if the forms it takes can sometimes go wrong. The Latin *caritas* translates as love. Ideas about solidarity and mutual aid, and looking after the weak, are central to a good society. Struggling against social inequality and injustice is not incompatible with emotional connection and moral commitment: after all, it was Che Guevara who wrote, 'The true revolutionary is guided by strong feelings of love'. Perhaps 'rights and charity' might be a better slogan or, in the words of the Old Testament prophet Micah, 'justice and mercy'. In this context, it is interesting that the Hebrew word for charity translates as righteousness, or justice. According to Simone Weil, 'The supernatural virtue of justice consists of behaving exactly as though there were equality when one is the stronger in an unequal relationship' (quoted in Gaita 2002: 202). Zygmunt Bauman quotes the Jewish philosopher Emmanuel Levinas, who argued, 'Charity is impossible without justice, but justice without charity is deformed' (Bauman, 1998: 49).

# Chapter 11

# Love, friendship, intimacy

## Introduction

When I helped research and write *The Sexual Politics of Disability* between 1994 and 1996, it was striking that issues of sexuality had a low profile in the British disability movement, and in the developing field of disability studies. It had been suggested by disabled feminists such as Jenny Morris (1993b) that disability studies was reproducing the same old academic problem, of talking about people, when in reality it was relevant only to men. However, we felt that something else was going on. The divide between the public and the private, which feminists had also identified, was the key factor explaining the neglect of issues of sex and identity within disability politics. That is, the public lives of disabled men and women were up for analysis, for discussion, and for campaigning. The demand for an end to discrimination in education, employment, etc. was all about making personal troubles into public issues. But the private lives of disabled women and men were not seen as being equally worthy of concern. It has to be remembered that the social model emerged in the 1970s, when the notion of the personal as political was only just emerging from the women's movement, and in Britain, where sexual conservatism was the norm.

Partly, this is undoubtedly about prioritisation. Ending poverty and social exclusion comes higher up the list of needs than campaigning for a good sex life, and for access to bars, restaurants and clubs. I think the neglect may also be to do with the ways in which the disability movement in Britain consciously tapped into the tradition of labour movement organising, and adopted the paradigms of trades unionism and socialism, rather than the paradigms of consciousness raising and feminism. The UPIAS tendency, adopting a leftist approach, overcame the Liberation Network tendency, adopting a feminist and personal growth approach. Male, instrumental, public, rational and material concerns were seen as more real and more pressing than domestic issues. Looking at some of the macho politics of disabled direct action, and at some of the confrontationalism and anger and bitterness displayed by activists also gives some clues as to why relationships and intimacy and child-rearing may not have been on the agenda.

Third, perhaps sexuality, for disabled people, has been an area of distress and exclusion for so long that it was sometimes easier not to consider it, than to engage with everything from which so many were excluded. Talking about sex and love relates to acceptance on a very basic level – both acceptance of oneself, and acceptance by significant others – and forces people to confront things which are very threatening, given the abusive and isolated lives of many disabled people. As Anne Finger suggests,

> Sexuality is often the source of our deepest oppression; it is also often the source of our deepest pain. It's easier for us to talk about – and formulate strategies for changing – discrimination in employment, education, and housing than to talk about our exclusion from sexuality and reproduction.
>
> (Finger, 1992: 9)

My colleagues Kath Gillespie-Sells and Dominic Davies and I sought to fill that gap with the research which led to our book *The Sexual Politics of Disability* (1996). We talked to disabled people about their experiences with sex, love and intimacy. They talked to us about their body image, and about how they challenged prevailing notions of normality. They talked about how they identified differently as men and women, straight and gay, because of the intersection of discourses of gender, sexuality and disability. Many of them talked about their sexual lives, and some about their experiences of abuse and pain. In our work, we aimed to replace what we saw as a medical model of disabled sexuality – dominated by erectile disfunction, movement limitations and other incompetencies – with a social model of disabled sexuality, which highlighted the barriers which our respondents faced. For example, our respondents talked about negative attitudes, barriers and self-esteem.

Re-evaluating this work, I believe that we did not go far enough. First, by accepting a convenient distinction between impairment and disability, and focusing almost exclusively on disabling barriers, we failed adequately to engage with the issue of bodies and diversity. Second, by making sexuality our primary concern, we failed to understand that intimacy is perhaps a greater priority for disabled people. Sexuality is an important form of intimacy, and modern Western societies are fascinated with sexual acts and sexualised bodies. But friendship and acceptance are more fundamental than sex. Despite the implication given by much of the media and popular culture, sex may be comparatively unimportant to a wide section of the population. From a life course perspective, sexual desire appears to play a major part in life between the age of puberty and midlife: perhaps three decades out of a possible seventy or eighty years. Of course, children are in many ways sexual beings, and it is offensive and inaccurate to see older people as asexual. Yet sexuality is undoubtedly different at different stages of the life course. Moreover, even during the peak period of sexuality, many individuals and relationships are not dominated by sex. Leonore Tiefer (1995) cites a historic study in *New England Journal of Medicine*. A survey of 100 self-defined 'happy' couples found that there was some sort of arousal or orgasm dysfunction in the majority of cases but that the couples considered themselves happy both sexually and nonsexually nonetheless (Frank *et al.*, 1978). It has been well-observed that frequency and importance of sexual activity declines as a relationship continues and matures, and other ways of relating become more important. But whereas sex is not always a priority, for almost all human beings the need for intimacy, companionship, and acceptance remains central from birth to death. People can survive, even flourish, without sex, but the majority of individuals would be desolate without friendship.

## The importance of friendship

Humans are social animals. There are some rare people who seek solitude and shun company. Some people have different ways of relating, for example those on the autistic spectrum. But most human beings seek company, recognition and acceptance, and without them life can be bleak, tedious and lonely. Friendship is important for emotional, practical and even medical reasons. Ray Pahl, the sociologist who pioneered the study of friendship, talks about the importance of 'social convoy', referring to the group of linked individuals who make their way through life:

> The accumulation of supporting experiences of various forms eventually leads individuals to feel securely that they are capable and competent people and that they can be confident in knowing that there are significant others who believe in them, who love them and who can be counted on in a crisis. Having this social support empowers people to live more effectively and, indeed, more healthily and for longer.
>
> (Pahl, 2000: 149)

Communities and networks are important not just because they make people feel happy and connected. Networks play a number of other functions as well as emotional support: instrumental aid (lifts, childcare, loans, finding work), appraisal (evaluating a problem or solution) and monitoring (Pescosolido, 2001: 472).

Research has linked lack of social support to adverse medical conditions. There is evidence that more diverse social networks are associated with resistance to illness. Separated and divorced people have higher mortality from certain diseases than married people (Pahl, 2000: 145). Socially isolated people die at two or three times the rate of people with a network of social relationships and sources of emotional support (Brunner, 1997). It is not clear how these mechanisms operate, but possibly psychological distress causes immunological changes which cause vulnerability to disease. It is known that cortisol, the hormone released in situations of stress, has bad effects on the heart and brain.

Friendship is not a simple matter. There are different sorts of friendship, and the social meaning and form of friendship has probably been different at different historical times and in different places. Moreover, different people do friendship differently: for example, male friendships typically are based on shared activities, whereas women's friendships typically are based on communication. In general, women seem to be better at friendship and interaction than men (Traustadóttir, 1993). In terms of the benefits provided, it has been suggested that there are two types of friends. First, there is the intimate friend with whom one shares private experience and emotions. This type of friendship can be a deep and caring bond, based on trust, liking, and probably a history of shared experiences. Intimate friends may not see each other frequently, but are there when needed. People may not have very many intimate friends, perhaps only two or three. Second, there are friends who are there for company and sociability. This is what is meant by a social life – friends who are available to do things with. Someone may need a large number of such friends, to maximise the chance that a friend is on hand at the time they're looking to socialise. Both types of friendship might characteristically provide practical help from time to time – for example, assistance or advice. And reciprocality is a necessary feature of friendship – each serves a function for the other, and there is give and take in the relationship.

In the twenty-first century, friends play a greater role than in previous points in human history. A century ago, we would have been socially and culturally determined by our family. Fifty years ago, this role would have been played by our work and career. Now it is the people we do things with that count. Developing rich and varied social connections and having friends is a hidden but vital dimension of society; 'in order for a citizen to be fully engaged in a good society, access to material resources is not enough: access to psychological resources is also necessary' (Pahl: 164).

## Disabled people and isolation

If friendship offers benefits which are medical and practical as well as emotional and social, then this is another reason why friendship should be particularly important to disabled people. Disabled people often have more difficulties than non-disabled people in dealing with both their bodies and health, and the environments and systems which they have to negotiate. They rely more on others to provide assistance on a day-to-day basis, and they may be more vulnerable to medical complications.

Yet while disabled people may have greater need of friends, they are less likely to be well integrated into networks and friendship circles. Disabled people differ from most other disadvantaged groups because they experience significantly greater isolation and loneliness. For working class and minority ethnic people, their neighbourhood will usually provide community. Moreover, the family may be a haven in a heartless world, where there are others who share the experience and who can provide role models. Women will also often be able to find role models, friends and supporters amongst female family and friends. Lesbian and gay people may find families and neighbourhoods threatening and isolating. Yet, for many, networks and subcultures can provide alternatives, particularly in urban areas. Some gay and lesbian people find their identity and their community in the commercial gay scene. Others turn to alternative communities or create 'families of choice' (Weeks et al., 2001) as an alternative to their local neighbourhoods or biological families.

By contrast, disabled people may not know any other disabled people in their family, neighbourhood or wider community. They may find it difficult to identify as disabled. They may be excluded from social settings. Prejudice, ignorance and hostility may create barriers which prevent connecting to strangers or make entering public spaces an ordeal (Watson, 2003). Disabled people may lack the energy or skills or resources to socialise. Community care has ensured that most people with impairments live in local neighbourhoods, not in segregated institutions, but many disabled people remain effective prisoners in their own homes. This may be because of environmental barriers, lack of money, feelings of vulnerability, or problems with mobility. It is known that older people are at risk of losing social contact and intimacy, but disabled people may also experience these difficulties. Reviewing two decades of literature on community-based services, Traustadóttir (1993) concludes that most disabled people continue to be isolated, lonely and have few friends. This disconnection may be more likely at particular times of the life course (Priestley, 2004) or for certain groups of disabled people.

For example, families which have a disabled member tend to be socially isolated. Parents may be struggling to survive on low incomes without sufficient services, and may not have time to support their disabled child to develop friendships. Evidence from social research with disabled children suggests that isolation from the peer group is a major issue for many young people with impairments (Priestley *et al.*, 1999; Skär, 2003). Some children may travel long distances to schools which can provide facilities for them, whether segregated or mainstream. The consequence is that they may lack friends in their own neighbourhoods. Many disabled children spend most of their time with adults. These may be their own parents, or special needs assistants in school, or other carers and therapists and support workers. Because they are always accompanied by adults they are denied access to the social world of children, and they may be unable to take part in age-appropriate activities and express the typical resistance of children and young people. Research shows that many disabled children have few or no friends. They may have 'hi friends', but not genuine intimates. For example, Huurre and Aro's 1998 study of adolescents with visual impairment found that they often had less friends than their peers and were more likely to report loneliness and low self-esteem. Karl Atkin and Yasmin Hussain (2003) found that young Asian disabled people were isolated and lacked networks. For example, asked about leisure, Shakeel replied, 'Spare time? I think every day is spare time for me' (Atkin and Hussain, 2003: 169), and Nasira told them, 'I don't have any friends because I don't go anywhere . . . They don't want me to come round because I'm disabled, you see, they don't want to know me' (Atkin and Hussain, 2003: 169).

Aitchison (2003) found that the young disabled people he researched with spent more of their leisure time in solitary and home-based pursuits such as watching television, listening to music, playing computer games. On average, his fifteen respondents had only one visit with a friend in the study fortnight. Pippa Murray's survey of 100 disabled teenagers found that most described lives as tainted by isolation, loneliness and exclusion (Murray, 2002). Lack of appropriate support – transport and personal assistance – was the major barrier to participation. Whereas professionals thought leisure opportunities were valuable ways of developing life skills and independence, young people's goal was friendship.

People with mental illness are another group of disabled people who are particularly likely to be isolated. For many people with mental illness, the community may be seen as frightening and lonely (Lester and Tritter, 2005). It may be difficult for people to sustain relationships, both because of the prejudice and fear associated with mental illness, and also because of the impact of mental illness on behaviour. People with psychosis are three times more likely to be divorced than the general population (Meltzer *et al.*, 2002). A recent survey of 3,000 people with severe mental illness found that even among those who had contact with support organisations, a quarter had no or very little involvement with communitiy activities (Pinfold, 2004). In four out of ten cases, the social networks of people with mental illness were limited to other people using or working in the mental health services. Eighty-four per cent of people with mental illness felt isolated, as opposed to 29 per cent of the general population.

People with learning difficulties also face problems with friendship. After de-institutionalisation, they may be present in the community, but not participating in it. Often, people with learning difficulties are isolated in subgroups of professional workers, and peers with learning difficulties. One study found that only one in three people using learning disability services had even one non-disabled friend (Robertson *et al.*, 2001). In their study of people living in supported accommodation in northern England, Emerson and McVilly (2004) found that 81 per cent of people with learning difficulties wanted to have more friends, and 65 per cent wanted a 'best friend' relationship. While 65 per cent had engaged in friendship activities with another person with learning difficulties, and 25 per cent with a friend who did not have learning difficulties, the median number of friendship activities over a four-week period was two. The researchers concluded that it was the setting, not the characteristics of the individual, which determined the level of social activity. Research about the accommodation goals of people with learning difficulties indicates that access to social networks of family and friends are vital aspects of living arrangements (Barr *et al.*, 2003). Respondents prioritised having privacy in their homes, but also feared being alone.

Other groups within the disabled population may not experience this degree of social exclusion. For example, people with restricted growth usually do not experience cognitive limitations, are able to work or participate in society, and often resist identification as disabled. Yet my team's ongoing research with people with restricted growth in the North of England has found a different social profile to the general population: out of 63 respondents at the time of writing, 55 per cent were single, compared to 30 per cent of the general population. Only 39 per cent were or had been married, compared to 69 per cent of the general population. While 12 per cent of the general population live alone, 30 per cent of our respondents lived alone. It would be wrong to conclude that all restricted growth adults are therefore lonely and isolated, but the data is suggestive of a group who may have less social contact than their non-disabled peers.

Even where disabled people have friends and companions, they may find it harder to experience everyday intimacies which non-disabled people take for granted. This is not just a matter of having children or having a family life, important though these issues are. Many experience frustrations and difficulties with communication, which cannot simply be attributed to oppression, but also arises from the very real problems in understanding some people with speech impediments. Some disabled adults experience little physical contact with others. Their body may usually be experienced in terms of pain, restriction and lack of control. The main occasion when others touch their body is when carers or personal assistants or professionals lift and handle them in daily living situations, or for medical interventions.

How can the isolation and loneliness of some disabled people be explained? It would be misleading to conclude that this was an inevitable outcome of having an impairment. However, neither is it simply a matter of social oppression. Wider societal trends, the particular barriers faced by disabled people, and the social predicament of impairment all contribute to the problem.

## The decline of community and struggle for connection

Western societies became increasingly individualised and atomised during the twentieth century, as traditional ties of family, religion and community declined. A range of social, economic and demographic factors reduced the strength of networks of kin, friends and community. For example:

1   Families are smaller and more dispersed.
2   Organised religion is a minority experience: social networks built around religion are less common.
3   People are more mobile, leaving their community of origin to attend higher education, and often relocating several times during their lives to find work.
4   Pressure of careers means that working age people are less likely to have time to dedicate to community activities. Because more women work, fewer people are exclusively home-makers.
5   Non face-to-face interaction – through telephones and internet – and passive forms of leisure – television and other multimedia – may have taken over from unmediated social engagement for many people. Rather than using the same local shops and services, and developing relationships with staff, people may drive to out of town shopping centres, where transactions are usually anonymous.

These factors, to varying degrees, erode continuity and interconnection. None of these changes make friendship impossible, and of course friendship in many ways has never been more important. These factors may contribute to changes in the form of friendship as much as to the decline of friendship. For example, people may make friends quickly – for example through work, or parenting networks – but move on equally quickly. People may not know their geographical neighbours, or take the time to make friends in their local communities, because they are connected to networks of interest. By contrast, in the past communities were based on long-term and stable familiarity and shared activities within localities. The anthropologist Mary Douglas differentiates between strong ties and weak ties:

> Strong ties are best for certain dependent categories of the population such as infants, elderly people, the handicapped and the chronically infirm. But strong ties broken are hard to mend: it is not easy to foster them at the right phase in the life cycle and to loosen them at other times. Weak ties on the other hand, appeal to our cultural bias in favour of an open society.
>
> (quoted Pahl 2000: 159)

All of these wider social factors make isolation and disconnection a problem for many people, not just non-disabled people. But they particularly impact on disabled people. Community care has meant that most disabled people are living in the community, just as the concept of community has been eroded.

## Disability, friendship and social barriers

Developing friendships depends on having opportunities to meet people, and having the skills to develop and sustain friendships. If we are to avoid falling into the traditional mistake of viewing disabled lives as inevitably sad and tragic, it is also important to understand the role of social factors. This means seeking explanations for disabled people's isolation in terms of environmental and social barriers, including educational segregation, employment discrimination and inaccessible transport and social environments.

In *The Sexual Politics of Disability* we argued that while the social model has been used to highlight the failures of contemporary social organisation – the badly designed transport, the prejudiced attitudes (Keith, 1996), and the discriminatory employers which disable people – it needs also to be used to show that the problem of disability and sexuality is not an inevitable outcome of our bodily differences. It is not because people cannot walk, or cannot see, or because they lack feeling in this or that part of the body that disabled people have sexual problems. As we argued, the problem of disabled sexuality is not how to do it, but who to do it with. The barriers to the sexual expression of disabled people are primarily to do with the society in which they live, not the bodies with which they are endowed. For example, many people find friends among the people with whom they study at school, college or university, and the people alongside whom they work. If disabled people are segregated in school, or excluded from further and higher education, and if they are twice as likely to be unemployed, then they will not only lack skills, opportunities and income, but they will also lack the social networks and self-esteem which successful participation in education and employment offers. If people lack money, they will be unable to buy drinks and meals, or tickets to films and other cultural events, even assuming that the venues for these activities are physically accessible.

Social and educational interventions to overcome social exclusion may well have paradoxical impacts on the inclusion and friendship opportunities of disabled people. For example, it has been suggested above that the presence of special needs assistants and other non-disabled helpers may lead to disabled children being excluded from peer groups, or finding it harder to reach out and make friends. Paradoxically, residential institutions and special schools were often places of security and friendship for disabled people, despite the problems of segregation, disempowerment and abuse in many settings. Edgerton (1984) showed how hidden subcultures in institutions emphasise sociability, harmony and self-esteem. Having the right to live independently in the community is a good principle, but in practice often translates into being isolated in a private home in the middle of a neighbourhood where there are few opportunities for networking or friendship. For many disabled or elderly people, attending a day centre or living in a group home may be preferable to being bored all day or living alone. Many disabled people are in the community, but not part of the community.

Disability services may not always recognise the problem. Promoting friendship opportunities might not be on their agenda. Workers may not see it as their job to help their clients with making friends. Disability services may focus on group activities, setting their clients apart from the mainstream, rather than on promoting opportunities on an individual basis. Many services are preoccupied with risk and protection, and may be concerned about exposing their clients to unstructured contact with the rest of the world. If people with learning difficulties start exploring their sexuality, for example, they may become vulnerable to abuse or exploitation.

The development of a disability rights movement may have benefits for disabled people in overcoming isolation and loneliness, as well as in other areas. For example, anti-discrimination legislation, removal of social and environmental barriers, accessible transport, more opportunities to participate in mainstream education and employment, and more economic resources all improve the quality of life of disabled people. As a result, people may have more social contacts, more opportunities, and more access to the mainstream world, all generating more inclusion. Second, disability rights approaches improve self-esteem, by relocating the problems of disabled people from the person themselves, to the oppressive society. Also, by showing how disabled people are oppressed, not simply unfortunate, perhaps the social model creates a moral imperative for non-disabled people to reach out to disabled people to try and overcome oppression and isolation. Third, the disability rights movement creates and sustains social networks, primarily between disabled people themselves (Campbell and Oliver, 1996). Coalitions, direct action protests and disability arts cabarets all offer opportunities for disabled people to link up with others. Subcultures, whether based on disability rights, or on shared impairment, can provide contexts for oppressed individuals to make friends and gain confidence.

While these outcomes should be valued, it could be argued that there may paradoxically be negative effects of the emergence of disability rights. For example, the disability movement may not be welcoming or inclusive to all disabled people, and there have been claims that minorities or those with particular impairments are not always equally represented or supported. Moreover, the rights discourse may encourage a political identity which is rejecting of non-disabled people, and promotes hostile and self-segregating responses. Gaining more disabled friends may sometimes be at the cost of abandoning those non-disabled acquaintances or family members who are seen as patronising and inappropriate in their response to disability. Of course, this may not be a negative outcome: fewer, better friends who contribute to self-esteem rather than putting you down might be preferable.

A social model analysis of the lack of friendship and intimacy in the lives of disabled people cannot fully account for this persistant and neglected problem. By definition, it is a social not a biological phenomenon. But it is not simply a matter of discrimination. It is partly about the predicament of impairment. Broader social changes have created a world in which disabled people are particularly disadvantaged, and the problems of being impaired are exacerbated. It is not just that disabled people and older people are disempowered and devalued. The social ecology of contemporary living has less space for those who may be able to contribute little to reciprocal relationships. The dominance of secularism, individualism and consumerism may accord little priority to helping those who are isolated and excluded.

## Achieving social interaction

Interaction between disabled and non-disabled people can be difficult for a range of reasons. Some of these are to do with the disabled person themselves. Some impairments make social relations more difficult. For example, people with speech impairments may be hard to understand (Paterson and Hughes, 1999). Deaf people may rely on sign language for communication, which many hearing people are unfamiliar with, or may have limited confidence with. Deafened or hard of hearing people may become very isolated as a result of difficulties of communicating with others. Most non-disabled people may not know how to go about communicating with a deaf-blind person. Some people with learning difficulties may also have little spoken language, sometimes relying on Makaton. In all these cases, relying on an interpreter may create a strained interaction. With familiarity and goodwill and patience, communication may become easier. But it may always be an effort for both parties to maintain a conversation.

In other cases, there may be no overt communication barrier, but interaction is still difficult. For example, people with learning difficulties may not behave conventionally or understand the subtleties of body language and ironic banter. People with mental health issues or cognitive impairment may lack insight, become anxious or suspicious, or otherwise interact in unusual ways. They may forget previous conversations or social contact. In the case of people with visual impairment, it may be difficult to initiate contact, or to communicate non-verbal cues. The lack of eye contact may be disconcerting for people unfamiliar with visually impaired people. In other cases, physical difference or deformity may be very distracting. As Erving Goffman (1968a) described, the effect of stigma is to undermine the possibilities of interaction, at least at the outset. It is difficult always to attribute these impairment effects to oppression or discrimination, rather than to social embarrassment and unfamiliarity. As Lenney and Sercombe (2002: 16) observe, 'the dynamics at work when people with disabilities interact with others are complex and contradictory'.

Impairment does not need to determine the outcome of interactions. After all, many people with highly visible impairments or communication difficulties manage social interactions very successfully. But, on average, such impairments do contribute to the social isolation of many disabled people. Those who achieve interaction do so by what Fred Davis (1964) called 'normalizing': going more than halfway, by enabling the non-disabled person to go beyond their preoccupation with the impairment, and finding what they both have in common (Fisher and Galler, 1988: 173). Skill and confidence is required if disabled people are to manage this move. Those who overcome social barriers often do so because their impairments are compensated by other factors. For example, they may enjoy cultural advantages of race, gender or status, or have resilient or gregarious personalities.

However, more often, because of the experience of both impairment and discrimination, and perhaps also because of the past experience of difficult communication, disabled people may lack confidence and self-esteem. For example, people with acquired brain injury may feel that their sense of identity has been taken away by their impairment (Sherry, 2002) . People who have been institutionalised all their lives may not have a strong sense of individuality or autonomy. In general, disabled people may have internalised negative messages from significant others, or from society in general, and believe themselves to be incompetent or invalid or undesirable. Alternatively, they may be angry and hostile about their situation, resenting the way they are treated, and unwilling to overlook actual or perceived slights from others (Keith, 1996). Both of these are understandable reactions to the difficulties of impairment and disability, but neither are conducive to comfortable relations with others.

Of course, it is important to note that the attitudes and behaviour of non-disabled people are a major factor in the extent to which disabled people are isolated or integrated into networks and communities (Keith, 1996; Tregaskis, 2004a). For example, there are various reasons why non-disabled people may be unwilling to make the effort to communicate with or associate with disabled people. If disabled people are segregated from non-disabled people, then lack of familiarity may generate fear and prejudice. Ignorance and lack of social skills might make it difficult for non-disabled people to overcome communication barriers or cope with unusual behaviour. Cultural representation of disabled people as asexual and uncool is unlikely to encourage non-disabled people to reach out to include disabled people in leisure or social activities. Because of their own insecurity, many people want to be associated with successful and high-achieving people: disabled people may be seen as incompetent, and as discrediting people to be around. If disabled people seem to be distressed or suffering, then this may be uncomfortable to non-disabled people who try to avoid the difficult aspects of life. Because a relationship with a disabled person may be perceived as asymmetrical, it may be assumed that the non-disabled person will not derive any personal benefit from the relationship. Finally, those who are willing to look past these issues and reach out to disabled people may not want to get into a caring role. This may particularly structure women's responses; 'Because women are assigned the roles of nurturer, helper, and healer, getting to know someone with a disability may seem to imply that the non-disabled woman must automatically become a caretaker' (Fisher and Galler, 1988: 76). At the extreme, there may be fear of fostering a relationship of dependency, where the disabled person makes excessive or continuing demands which the non-disabled person is unwilling or unable to fulfil (DisAbility Services, n.d.: 16).

However, these negative responses are not the whole picture. There are many individuals who are willing to associate with disabled people, reach out to them, and include them in their lives and communities. When people become friends with disabled people, the salience of the impairment may diminish: the disabled person becomes 'delabelled' (Taylor and Bogdan, 1989: 32) and accepted as normal, and the relationship can become reciprocal. Traustadóttir (1993) argues that women are overrepresented in social networks of disabled people, and play an important role in providing social support. Women seem to be more accepting than men of disabled people. Men may find it difficult to provide assistance to disabled friends, or may be ill at ease with emotional intimacy.

Following Taylor and Bogdan's 1989 work on the sociology of acceptance, we can identify several reasons why non-disabled people put in the extra effort and reach out to disabled people. First, people are bonded by the family relationships they have with disabled people: 'The family would not be the same family without the disabled family member' (Taylor and Bogdan, 1989: 27). Parents and siblings of disabled people who contributed to the AnSWeR website (www.antenataltesting. info) show how their lives are enriched by disabled family members, and the commitment they have to them.

Second, there are actually major benefits to associating with disabled people. People like and enjoy the company of disabled people, as this respondent indicated – 'I really like spending time with him. Why? Because we both have active imaginations, we're artistic, share the same sense of humour, love chocolate, and like good coffee on Sunday mornings' (Taylor and Bogdan, 1989: 32). Disabled people may be enjoyable and amusing, and their company may form an alternative to the more competitive, status-oriented or stressful social relations in the mainstream world. For example, it is often suggested that people with learning difficulties are more open, generous, trusting and lighthearted than non-disabled people. They may have a sense of humour and a joy in life which is very valuable (Vanier, 1999).

Third, non-disabled people may be motivated by the benefits for their own sense of self which they derive from reaching out to less fortunate people. They may get a sense of purpose in life. They may feel that here they are doing something rewarding. They may feel that they are better people as a result. They may in fact be socially valued by their community or society because of their charitable work. As a result of their work with disabled people, their own self-esteem may be enhanced (Wuthnow, 1991).

Fourth, people may make the effort to include and support disabled people for ideological reasons: they may have a religious commitment, and therefore believe that the role of a Good Samaritan or good neighbour or charitable person is desirable, is part of their religious faith, or may result in reward in the afterlife. Alternatively, they may have a sense of social solidarity for political or humanist reasons, and believe that it is their duty to include others and to overcome oppression: for example, the women's movement explicitly fostered friendships between women, and friendships between women from different backgrounds (Fisher and Galler, 1988). People who work professionally with disabled people may extend this into friendships with disabled people in their personal lives.

Reciprocity seems to be an important element in proper friendship. This may remain a problem, even when disabled people are skilled in reaching out, and non-disabled people are motivated to make and stay friends. While personal assistance and better services may make disabled people less reliant on their friends, there will always be situations in which help is required. Disabled people may minimise their needs, in order to avoid asking for help from a friend and unbalancing the relationship. Reciprocity may also apply to topics for conversation – for example, censoring of conversations about sexuality and childbearing and even disability itself has been reported by disabled women (Fisher and Galler, 1988: 183). Non-disabled people may feel guilt about not sharing the limitations or difficulties of their disabled friend. All this complicates interaction, and sometimes affects the possibility for emotional openness and exchange.

Sometimes, friendships between disabled and non-disabled people occupy an ambiguous space. In describing the friendship between Michelle, a non-disabled woman, and Susan, a woman with significant learning difficulties, Traustadóttir (2000) shows Michelle used the language of work as well as the language of love. Whereas the ideal was for their relationship to be a true and mutual friendship, in practice the day-to-day reality was of Michelle having to work hard to establish and develop their companionship. Normal friendships are usually homogenous and balanced. But these types of worked-at friendships do not conform to the culturally dominant view of friendship. Here, the rewards are not reciprocation and mutual support, but the satisfaction of making someone else happier and more included, and playing a socially valued role.

## How can isolation and loneliness be overcome?

If isolation and loneliness cannot simply be attributed to oppression, it is difficult to see how barrier removal alone could entirely solve the problem. A society with strong anti-discrimination legislation and good access would certainly be one in which disabled people were more socially engaged, but not all disabled people would automatically be included. Particular groups may be at particular risk of isolation – for example, people with learning difficulties or mental health issues – and particular points in the life course may be difficult for disabled people – for example, adolescence. Social welfare agencies and social movements need to understand these issues, and make a positive contribution to fostering social networks and community for and with disabled people.

### Staff

Staff can be pivotal in promoting inclusion and friendship. Taxi drivers, carers, nursing and medical professionals do emotional work, providing friendship and validation, not just the obvious practical tasks. Many disabled people rely on their personal assistants to provide companionship as well as practical help. A traditional stress on professionalism and distance needs to give way to what Traustadóttir calls 'commitment and involvement' (1993: 122). Some currents in disability rights discourse risk neglecting these aspects of the helping role. Non-disabled people, and professionals in particular, can be seen as potential exploiters or abusers, rather than potential allies. Sometimes, personal assistants are treated as servants, and the psycho-emotional aspects of the role are downplayed, as I discuss elsewhere in this book.

### Services

Services could be audited to explore whether they increase or decrease the isolation of disabled people. Rather than solely focusing on inclusion, provision should also aim to build shelter and interconnectedness. For example, special needs assistants in classrooms often tend to increase children's isolation, even if they succeed in meeting other needs. Imagination may be needed to deliver support in ways which do not single out the recipient, or exclude them from other valuable interactions. New initiatives should be assessed in terms of whether they impact on possibilities of friendship and intimacy, helping build connections. For example, relying on email or telephone rather than face-to-face communication may be efficient, but reduces opportunities for social contact; 'While the screen may open the user to new worlds, it may also serve to deepen isolation and prevent acquisition of the skills and confidence required to conduct relationships in the everyday world' (Seymour and Lupton, 2004: 302). For other groups, providing online discussion opportunities may build connections and promote mutual support. For example, people with rare conditions may find comradeship in national and international list-servs such as the Shortlist e-group for people with restricted growth. People with communication or social interaction issues may find online groups easier to negotiate than face-to-face gatherings.

There is potential for staff to do more to help friendship. For example, people who work with and for disabled people should promote a community development model of service provision, looking for opportunities for their clients to make connections and engage in social activities. Rather than only group activities, staff could facilitate individualised social activities for clients. A proactive and imaginative worker could stimulate ideas, facilitate oppportunities, and act as an entrepreneur, creating connections based on shared interests. The Metro Access workers in Victoria, Australia, seem to be playing exactly this role, looking at how mainstream community organisations and activities can accommodate participation by disabled people.

### Voluntary groups

Voluntary groups in the disability community create possibilities of friendship and companionship, as well as having instrumental value in campaigning or providing services. Disability rights groups, self-advocacy groups and more traditional self-help groups bring isolated people together and make spaces for friendships to grow. Cultural projects also play a role. Examples include the network of arts studios where people with mental health issues can drop in and spend time. The staff are professional artists, rather than care workers, and provide company, as well as fostering creativity. Theatre groups for people with learning difficulties (such as Olla in Sweden and The Lawnmowers in Gateshead, UK) can enhance confidence, challenge negative attitudes, and provide meaningful social activity. Disability arts cabaret nights and nightclubs for people with learning difficulties (for example, the Krocodile Klub and the Big Snapper) offer spaces where disabled people can socialise with others on their own terms (Price and Barron, 1999).

### Friendship circles

Various initiatives have tried to provide a framework upon which genuine friendship can develop. In the absence of spontaneous social networks and traditional communities, artifical ways of creating companionship and friendship for disabled people need to be explored (Abraham, 1989). These include friendship circles (Perske, 1988) and 'bridge-building'. For example, Circles of Support (Gold, 1999) are networks of non-disabled people which provide friendship opportunities for a disabled child or adult. Often these have been organised by the parents of young people with learning difficulties with the aim of promoting the inclusion of their child. However, sometimes these friendships do not outlast the duration of the group meetings. Moreover, there is a tension between the hope for 'true friendship' and the danger of creating a support service which stigmatises the disabled person at the centre – 'We must guard against merely creating another generation of "professionals" and "clients", with the former group seen as perpetually competent, and the latter, perpetually needy' (Van Der Klift and Kunc, 1994: 3). Providing too much help can itself be disempowering. Friendship is an elusive thing which cannot easily be engineered.

## Training

It has been suggested that people with learning difficulties or other cognitive impairments may benefit from training so that they can learn how to make friends. For example, programmes can teach friendship skills to adolescents with high functioning autism and Asperger syndrome (Duffield, 2001). This approach may seem patronising. However, learning how to communicate, how to be sensitive to boundaries, how to overcome jealousy or possessiveness, are all complex skills which are gained through experience and through watching others. Arguably, people can be helped to develop and practice these skills through role play for example, which facilitates mutual understanding and appropriate behaviour, and helps with conflict resolution. The danger is that a focus on skills means that people spend the time learning, not getting out and making friends. When the DisAbility Services Branch of the Department of Human Services, Victoria commissioned research to investigate social networks among people with a cognitive impairment, and how these could be enhanced, their report focused on social inclusion, not just skills development. A major emphasis was on accessing communities based on shared interests – for example, sports and pets – rather than geographical proximity. The conclusion of their research was that a focus on friendship could bring about a major shift in the provision of services for people with learning difficulties.

## Education

In order to become friends, non-disabled people need to be able to learn about disability, both in general, and in terms of the specific individual with whom they are engaging. Ignorance and fear – including fear of doing or saying the wrong thing – are barriers to social interaction (Lenney and Sercombe, 2002: 17). Inclusion of disabled people in schools establishes familiarity between disabled and non-disabled people. Education about impairment and disability, and by disabled people, may challenge myths and establish ways of being together. Ultimately, disabled people may still need to explain and to educate their non-disabled colleagues and friends about what their own impairment means, and where accommodation will have to be made. This requires patience and commitment and communication from both sides.

# Conclusion

In the course of writing this chapter, I looked at the index of half a dozen recent disability studies texts (Campbell and Oliver, 1996; Barnes and Mercer, 2003;

Swain *et al.*, 2003; Swain *et al.*, 2004; Barnes and Mercer, 2004; Barnes *et al.*, 2002). There was minimal discussion of friendship, sexuality, or loneliness. Most of the research which has been done on friendship and disability has been restricted to issues for people with learning difficulties. Although there has been a scattering of interesting initiatives in the field of sexuality – for example, research on facilitated sex (Earle, 1999), work with lesbian and gay people with learning difficulties (Abbott and Mitchell, 2005), and the 2005 *Disability Now* sex survey – it seems that none of the leading authors in British disability studies has built on the work we started in 1996. Equally, mainstream studies of intimacy and friendship do not usually attend to particular issues for disabled people (e.g. Jamieson, 1998). The British disabled feminist Liz Crow wrote:

> I've always assumed that the most urgent Disability civil rights campaigns are the ones we're currently fighting for – employment, education, housing, transport etc., etc., and that next to them a subject such as sexuality is almost dispensable. For the first time now I'm beginning to believe that sexuality, the one area above all others to have been ignored, is at the absolute core of what we're working for . . . It's not that one area can ever be achieved alone – they're all interwoven, but you can't get closer to the essence of self or more 'people-living-alongside-people' than sexuality, can you?
>
> (Crow, 1991: 9)

While endorsing Crow's point, it seems to me to be a broader and deeper problem than that of sexuality alone. Prior to sexual expression is the problem of basic companionship, conversation, and togetherness. Steve Taylor and Robert Bogdan (1989: 34) call for a sociology of acceptance: research into what can foster connection, how relationships can be supported, and how both disabled and non-disabled people can be enabled to form relationships with each other. This agenda should be an important part of disability studies.

Policies which took the intimacy and friendship needs of disabled people seriously would see support as more diverse than simple daily living tasks. Clearly, this could be controversial. Funding might be provided for disabled people to have massages, or even to buy sexual services. When paid help includes intimate bodily activities, then the potential for abuse or exploitation is increased – and the provider of services may be exploited, not just the recipient. But despite this danger, a clearly defined and well regulated system might go some way to meeting the less obvious physical and emotional needs of disabled people.

Trying to support inclusion and friendship opportunities for disabled people is complex and difficult. Different solutions each involve tensions and compromises. For example, the Camphill or L'Arche communities seem to provide safe and sheltered environments, where people with learning difficulties are supported within family structures, engage in work, and can have freedom to live normally. Yet this is achieved by creating a rather segregated and unusual rural village situation, in which very motivated non-disabled people live with a high proportion of people who need support (Vanier, 1999; Rawles, 2004). Equally, artificial ways of fostering connection may seem patronising. The skeleton of contact and exchange which such structures provide may not seem genuine or worthwhile. But over time, such relationships can develop into important and mutually satisfying connections. Moreover, to many people who benefit from volunteering schemes – particularly older people and people with learning difficulties – their benefits outweigh any anxieties about charity or paternalism which disability rights activists have sometimes expressed.

Traustadóttir (2000) warns against the idealism found in many rosy and inspirational stories of friendship between non-disabled people and people with learning difficulties. She shows how these relationships are in practice harder and more complex than they first appear, and are usually rather different from conventional mutually supportive friendships. There is a danger of over-romanticising the difficulties of enabling disabled people, particularly those with significant cognitive problems, to form true relationships and achieve intimacy.

While there has been considerable attention to the friendship needs of particular groups of disabled people – people with learning difficulties and with mental health issues in particular – it seems to me that community and connection is an issue for many others who have physical impairments, particularly those which affect communication or hearing. Older people, with and without impairments, are clearly also at risk of isolation. Moreover, in an atomised contemporary world, the benefit of initiatives to support disabled people may be experienced by non-disabled people too (Bates and Davis, 2004). The social gathering which supports the disabled individual gives something meaningful to the non-disabled participants, who may also feel lonely at times. The benefit of volunteering, to give another example, is in the fulfilment and meaning it provides to those who volunteer, as well as to those who receive support. Just as the isolation of disabled people is about wider social changes, not just the predicament of impairment, so the solutions to that isolation may have wider impacts beyond the world of disability.

# Chapter 12

# The role of non-disabled people in the world of disability

At the core of the politics of disability is the attempt by disabled people to take back control over their lives. Rather than non-disabled people taking decisions, speaking for, or otherwise dominating them, disabled people are asserting their ability and right to be independent. So central is the concept of 'nothing about us, without us' that Charlton (1998) uses it as the title of his study of the worldwide disability movement. In the process, the roles of many different groups of non-disabled people in the lives of disabled people are repudiated: parents; volunteers and carers; professionals; organisations which are not accountable to their users; researchers who seek to understand the experience of disability. This long-overdue move puts disabled people themselves at the centre of the definition of disability and appropriate responses to it (Branfield, 1999).

This principle of disabled leadership connects to the minority group conception of disability. Here, disabled people are seen as a distinct group in society, who are oppressed and marginalised. Growing out of this analysis, identity politics bolsters the self-esteem and pride of the minority community, and further separates the community of disabled people from non-disabled people. Disability is seen as a dominant marker or master status, something which serves to divide society into two mutually exclusive groups, disabled and non-disabled. This approach borrows from the radical feminist idea of sex class, and the polarity between men and women, and the dominance of patriarchy. It also borrows from concepts of race and ethnicity. Disabled people are seen in ethnic terms, as a group with their own culture, language and ways of being. Disabled people share certain historical experiences – segregated schooling, residential living, day centres, special transport, professional and hospital care – which create a shared sense of self, and a set of shared cultural references. Gill suggests that these separate experiences mean that only disabled people can understand disability. 'Non-disabled people, no matter how much they love us, do not know the inside experience of being disabled. Moreover they are in a position to escape the stigma' (Gill, 1994). While oppressive systems are rejected, the idea of creating and sharing a disability culture – based on pride and resistance, not shame and exclusion – has become increasingly powerful in western countries since the birth of the disability movement. Disability arts has advocated and celebrated this notion of a distinct disability culture.

Taking its lead from the political and cultural struggles for recognition, disability studies has encouraged researchers to put disabled people at the centre of the picture and to prioritise the voices of disabled people. This is a very welcome move. Whereas historically research and policy was dominated by proxies for disabled people (parents, carers, professionals), now it is the views of disabled people themselves which matter most. Rather than seeing disabled people as objects of care and concern, disabled people are seen as subjects, entitled to choices and inclusion. The ideal of emancipatory research suggests that the research agenda should be generated by disabled people, and that researchers – whether disabled or non-disabled – should be accountable to organisations of disabled people.

In this chapter I want to explore the role of non-disabled people in disability. My claim is that the commendable urge to put disabled people at the centre of analysis, politics and policy has sometimes led to a writing out of non-disabled people. For example, in Priestley's otherwise valuable summary of the life course of disabled people, the role of the parents of the disabled person, or their siblings, or their spouses or partners, or in turn their children, is nowhere properly considered, despite the extent to which disability also impacts in their lives (Priestley, 2004). It is as if the disabled person exists in a vacuum.

The effect of these processes is to overlook three important aspects of the disability issue. First, the onset of impairment can come at any point in the life course. Non-disabled people are always vulnerable to becoming impaired. Whereas the vast majority of people are born into the sex which they remain for the rest of their lives, many people are born free of significant impairment, but become impaired through accident, disease or the ageing process at a later stage of life. Some people have impairments in childhood, but grow up to become non-disabled adults. The boundary between disabled people and non-disabled people is permeable in a way that gender boundaries or ethnic boundaries usually are not.

Second, impairment/disability is only one part of the identity and experience of disabled people. It may not be the dominant factor in their lives, and other aspects of their identity may have greater salience for some or all of the time. For example, most people have multiple affiliations: they may be more likely to associate and self-define in terms of their sexuality, ethnicity, religion or gender than their impairment. In other words, they may feel they have more in common with other gay people or Muslim people, than with others who share their impairment but nothing else. Indeed, the impairment experience itself may be very different depending on context, culture and opportunity: simply having the same diagnosis may not mean having the same impairment/disability experience.

Third, non-disabled people are a necessary and desirable part of most disabled people's lives. Only the most separatist disabled activist chooses to socialise or work exclusively with other disabled people. Many disabled people are the only disabled person in their family, or their workplace. Often, their parents, siblings, partner, neighbours, workmates and friends may be largely non-disabled. Some people actively avoid associating with people who share their experience of impairment or disability. Rather than allowing impairment/disability to dominate their lives, they adopt a 'really normal' persona, disavowing their difference and seeking what connects them to non-disabled people, not what separates them. The insepara-bility of disabled from non-disabled people makes the disability experience more like that of women than that of ethnic minorities, and makes the notion of a separate disability identity problematic. Only in the case of Deaf people does an ethnic conception of disability begin to work.

Given the difficulties of separating, practically or conceptually, the lives of disabled people from non-disabled people, it seems striking that disability studies and disability activism has failed adequately to conceptualise or understand the roles of non-disabled people. There is a considerable focus on oppression, but less focus on partnership or alliance. It is necessary to understand the roles that non-disabled people play in the lives of disabled people, and to explore some of the ways that non-disabled people can grow better relationships in which disabled people are supported to have better and more included lives. Whether disabled people – or anyone else – can be truly autonomous is a difficult question. But they can certainly never be autarkic, or self-sufficient. This chapter will open up explorations in some of the different roles in which non-disabled people encounter and live alongside disabled people. There is no intention of denying that disabled people themselves also take up these roles, only to expand our thinking about the ways in which disability affects non-disabled people.

## Parents

When I first came to think about families and parents (Shakespeare, 2000), I thought it was important to challenge the traditional valuation of family support for disabled people. Whereas parents had previously been celebrated as altru-istic and nurturing, I pointed to the inequality, oppression and abuse which were sometimes a feature of the family, taking my lead from feminist critiques of patriarchal family forms. The following paragraph is taken from this earlier analysis.

The ideology of the family exerts a powerful influence on our understanding of helping, and it casts a long shadow over the contemporary arrangement of community care (Dalley, 1988). As feminists have shown, too much of community care rests ultimately on the unpaid caring work of women in the home, who are expected to be the natural carers of people who are chronically ill or impaired, or who are elderly. Care is seen to belong in the idealised nuclear family, while paid care is viewed as second best. So the emphasis of much social policy is on sustaining family care, and when voluntary agencies or the state provide residential care as an alternative to the family, it tends to reinforce the same model (Brechin *et al.* 1998). Yet, while family care and the 'normal home' are meant to be the ideal, social research and analysis also suggests we should be suspicious or cautious about what goes on in the domestic environment. Parental love and support, which we have been lead to expect as unlimited and unconditional, seems to be more unreliable than ideology claims.

This approach, which I took in 2000, echoes the tradition of disability rights thinking. Early independent living activists such as Simon Brisenden criticised the way that society relied on families to provide unpaid care, suggesting that 'It exploits both the carer and the person receiving care. It ruins relationships between people and results in thwarted life opportunities on both sides of the caring equation' (Brisenden, 1989: 218).

More recently, writers on mental health have shown how parents are part of the problem for many people who experience mental illness (see for example the role of 'expressed emotion', Leff, 2001). In one of the few disability studies discussions of parents, Dona Avery discusses the 'tragedy' stories which were deployed by the parents of disabled people who participated in her online discussions (Avery, 1999). She argues that there is a lack of attention to the experience of parents, and how this is influenced by 'the socially derived guilt of shame attached to disability' (Avery, 1999: 117). Avery calls for parents to resist stories which situate their disabled children as patients, and to adopt a minority group perspective rather than a medicalised one.

While accepting the importance of independent living and demedicalisation, I think there might be a danger of ignoring or undervaluing the role of parents. In stressing the negative aspect, there is a danger of giving an unbalanced picture, and failing to see all the good and hard work which parents of disabled children do. Parents are almost always the primary carers of disabled children: they help them through encounters with doctors and hospitals, they support them through education, and try to enable them to make a successful transition to adulthood. Parents also suffer when they see their child suffer. Jeni Harden's work with parents of young people with mental health problems shows how they feel responsible for their children, they try to solve their problems, and they feel anxious about their future (Harden, 2005). Karl Atkin and Yasmin Hussain found an ambivalence when they spoke to Asian parents:

> Parents were vital allies for their children. There is thus a constant tension in the parents' narratives as they try to make sense of their own sadness at having a disabled child, while at the same time wanting to ensure the best opportunities for their child.
>
> (Atkin and Hussain, 2003: 166)

Parents advocate for their children, if they are either too young or too impaired to speak for themselves, to help them get the services to which they are entitled. Dora Bjarnason argues that parents are crucial to the later trajectories of their disabled children – 'early parental decisions and family support systems will affect the claims of disabled persons to adulthood and his or her possibilities to be both heard and understood' (Bjarnason, 2002: 316).

The support of professionals is crucial in enabling parents to become effective supporters of their children. Bjarnason shows how parents swing between different responses to their situation: action, anomie, passive acceptance and reaction. Those who were able to take action, were able to help their adult disabled children join the mainstream and achieve independence.

Dan Goodley's work in the self-advocacy movement highlights this ambivalence about the role of parents (2003: 112): on the one hand, his research found that parents had been a source of strength for people with learning difficulties, pushing for mainstream schooling, giving them a positive sense of self. On the other hand, parents were seen as being unable to let go, as being over-protective. In any family, parenting is a difficult balancing act: it is not just disabled people who are critical of over-protectiveness and interference by parents in their lives.

Giving a more balanced account of the contribution of parents also highlights the way that impairment/disability impacts on non-disabled family members. Often, the demands of supporting a disabled child means that one parent cannot work, with consequent pressure on household income and possible interruption to career. In Britain and many other countries, inadequate resources and services available to support disabled children and young adults mean that in many ways it is the whole family which is disabled, not just the disabled person. Jane Brett discusses the problems in the relationship between parents of severely impaired children and professionals, arguing that parents are controlled and disempowered by professionals: she calls for an 'alliance model' to overcome these difficulties (Brett, 2002). The value of social model approaches has been in shifting the focus from having an impairment to being oppressed and excluded by disabling barriers. Where non-disabled parents and family members are also impacted by oppression and exclusion, there is a sense in which they too could be conceptualised as disabled (Dowling and Dolan, 2001).

## Carers

While disability rights activists may have played down the role of parents, carers have often received attention, but usually negative. For example, there has been a suspicion of the concept of carers' rights in the disability movement, and a fear that authorities and researchers will substitute speaking to carers for the often harder task of gathering the views of disabled people themselves. When I inter-viewed independent living activists, they told me that the best way to improve the rights of carers is to improve the rights of disabled people. One disabled respondent spoke bitterly about his local carers' organisation, which did not even have a fully accessible building: 'I wish I had kinder things to say about carers' organisations. I don't.' He went on to add, 'to my mind, the more you increase the rights of carers, the more you take them away from disabled people'. These perspectives were reflected in my book *Help* (2000), expressing scepticism about the caring industry, and fear that the very real problems of those who provide care can distract from and take priority over the rights of those who receive it.

For example, the Carers National Association was formed in 1986. A key 'moral entrepreneur' in the social construction of the concept of the carer was Jill Pitkeathley, whose book defined a carer as 'someone whose life is in some way restricted by the need to be responsible for the care of someone who is mentally ill, mentally handicapped, physically disabled or whose health is impaired by sickness or old age' (Pitkeathley, 1989: 11). This statement shows how the notion of the carer rests on the construction of the category of helpless person who requires care. The terminology used by Pitkeathley includes words such as 'dependent person', 'sufferers', 'heavily dependent person'. In stressing the problems of carers, Pitkeathley made totalising generalisations which stress the negative rather than the positive aspects of the relationship, and which reinforce the idea of the helped person as burden. For example, she suggests that carers experience isolation, being undervalued, fear, resentment, anger, guilt, embarrassment, role reversal, sense of loss, effects of emotional stress, strain on relationships, bereavement. Undoubtedly many do, but the effect is to blame the victim, and to ignore the structural causes of the difficulties facing carers.

The solutions proposed by Pitkeathley echo those feminist theorists of care who proposed institutionalisation and residential care (Dalley, 1988; Ungerson, 1987): for example, she talks about the need to move away from a nuclear family model towards a collectivist approach. Yet she did not consider the views and preferences of disabled and older people themselves. Again, she opposed the idea that direct payments to disabled people would solve the problem of unpaid and exploitative care: because of her overwhelming focus on the needs of the carer, she suggests that the money should go direct to them, not to the service users. Much of the philosophy, if not the financial suggestions, contained in Pitkeathley's book went into the 1995 Carers Act, which defined a carer as someone providing more than 20 hours' care per week.

For the disability movement, the key to solving the problem of care is to empower disabled people themselves (Morris, 1993b). For example, direct payments would allow disabled people to employ personal assistants rather than rely on unpaid care. Equally, given the contentious academic debates about the role of children as carers, proper personal assistance schemes would avoid this necessity.

Thinking about the role of non-disabled people as carers suggest the importance of reconciliation between the disability rights perspective and the perspective of carer advocates. For example, drawing on the work of Jenny Morris, Bill Bytheway and Julia Johnson (1998) analysed the social construction of 'carers', and challenged the perspective of the carers movement. Their work highlights the concept of 'caring systems' in which mutuality plays a key role, and concludes that care should be reconceived as a normal part of ordinary family and community life.

As I argue elsewhere in this book, independent living will never replace entirely the role of unpaid care by family members. Whether as parents of disabled children, partners or spouses of disabled adults, or children of disabled and elderly parents, non-disabled people will always play a role in supporting disabled people. While progressive social arrangements can diminish the social dependency experienced by people who cannot meet their own physical needs, the need for what feminist theorists call 'caring solidarity' will continue to be vital. The financial, social and personal impact on those who care for others also remains important. This illustrates the stake that non-disabled carers have in the disability debate: here, too, non-disabled people are disadvantaged and excluded as a consequence of impairment/disability. The challenge remains to improve the quality of life of both disabled people, and the non-disabled people who support them.

## Professionals

*clues about how social model advocates would see integration* ↓

Roles like personal assistant and advocacy worker are emerging and as yet are unprofessionalised. However, the existing professions – doctors, professions allied to medicine, social workers and psychologists – have traditionally played important roles in the lives of disabled people, and consequently have received considerable and usually critical attention from activists and academics.

Typical is the article by Ken Davis (1993) on 'the crafting of good clients', first published in *Coalition* in September 1990. Davis is scathing about the role of these 'professionals':

> There are lots of them, they have different titles and work for different agencies, and often we get a bit confused as to who they are. They learn about disability by doing courses and reading books. Some of them are given diplomas for doing this, so they can then prove how expert they are in disability matters. These paper qualifications help them get jobs and make careers out of our needs.
>
> (Davis, 1993: 197)

Davis goes on to describe such workers as 'professional disability parasites' (1993: 199). This style of analysis is continued by Michael Oliver, who suggested that the main beneficiaries of the NHS, for example, are the doctors and nurses who work for it (Oliver, 1991, 157), by Vic Finkelstein (1980), and by many others in the disability rights tradition. In America, Irving Zola concluded:

> As long as the deliverers of service are markedly different in gender, economic class and race from those to whom they offer services, as long as accessibility to medical care is a privilege rather than a right, as long as the highest income groups are health care professionals, as long as the most profit-making enterprises include the pharmaceuticals and insurance industries, society is left with the uncomfortable phenomen of a portion of its population, living and living well, off the sufferings of others and to some extent even unwittingly having a vested interest in the continung existence of such problems.
>
> (Zola, 1977: 66)

Again, my own analysis of professionals in *Help* (2000) followed this approach. Drawing on the medical sociology literature of Friedson (1970) and Illich (1977) I argued that professionals were in a position to define need, to define disabled people and others who received help, and to meet needs on their own terms.

I challenged notions of expertise, and the way that technical language was used to control and exclude. I criticised the way in which the training of medical professionals made them less able to empathise and communicate with disabled people (Fraser, 1992: 27; St Claire, 1986). I also suggested that one source of the problem was the polarisation between those who received professional care, and those who provided professional care. The historical exclusion of disabled people from the professions fuels the lack of understanding and mutual respect.

Re-evaluating the disability studies literature on professionals, again I suggest that there is an imbalance in these accounts. While many disabled people have suffered at the hands of professionals, there are many others who have had good accounts of professional care. Nor is it clear that the majority of professionals are motivated by a desire to control, exploit or profit from their patients and clients. The resentment and hostility expressed by many activists seems inappropriate and unconstructive. It is clear that good quality medical or therapeutic assistance is vital to many disabled people. Rather than rejecting professionalism, the disability rights community needs to find ways of working to improve the relationship between disabled people and the professionals who are meant to serve them.

Susan Deeley's 2002 research with professionals working with people with learning difficulties shows a dualism between those who adhere to the prevailing orthodoxy of normalisation, and those who challenge it in favour of a more paternalistic ideology. She alerts us to internal conflicts within professionalism, which may be as relevant as potential disputes between professionals and disabled people (or their parents). They also reflect gradually changing relationships in the care sector: it was older professionals who considered normalisation to be unrealistic and impractical, whereas newer staff had more progressive ideas. Research by Ingrid Helgøy et al. (2003) shows how professionals and service providers can take at least five different roles: the rehabilitator, who imposes their ideology, authority and skills; the servant, for example in the personal assistance role; the caregiver, for example in the role of home help or nurse, where there may be tension between the demands of the disabled person and the caregiver's own professional standards; the shock absorber, who intercedes between the welfare bureaucracy and frustrated disabled people, and shares the frustration of their clients; the lawyer, who acts as a street-level bureaucrat helping their clients work the system. Each of these different approaches leads to different relationships with the different possible roles of disabled people (super-normal, powerless and resigned, seeking control).

One way of challenging the tradition of domination is for more disabled people to enter the professions. In her research with disabled health and caring professionals, Sally French (1998) found that despite the barriers and obstacles they experienced, many disabled professionals felt they had the advantage of improved empathy, understanding and communication with their patients and clients. As more disabled people enter the professions, it is possible that the relationship between user and provider of help may change. Another way forward is for professional training and practice to recognise the rights and support the autonomy of disabled people. For example, many medical schools are now bringing in disabled people as tutors and lecturers to train future doctors. Valuing the life experience and expertise of disabled people could enable professional and patient to work together to find more appropriate solutions to health and care needs. The priority is to replace relations of domination with relations of partnership.

However, what is not going to change is the need for specialist expertise and interventions in the lives of many disabled people. Although not all disabled people are in need of professional support, having an impairment – or experiencing the social disadvantages often associated with impairment – makes disabled people more likely to use doctors, therapists and other professionals. This puts professionals in an important position in the disability field. Those who have made disability their life's work may have an insight into the problems and priorities for this population. A disabled individual may generalise from their own limited experience, while a professional may have a much broader knowledge of the impairment group. Indeed, many professionals have played important roles in developing self-help and advocacy groups for and with disabled people and their families: Goodley and Moore (2000: 880) applaud this radical professionalism, which promotes inter-dependence, focuses on capacity and takes a back seat. Nor is a professional's insight necessarily limited to, or skewed by, their disciplinary affiliation: many medical practitioners have independently realised that the problems of disabled people are primarily ones of participation and poverty, not illness and impairment (Colver, 2005).

## Support workers

Discussion of carers in disability literature is frequent and usually disparaging, because traditionally carers have sometimes taken away power, control and voice from the people they are meant to be supporting. As Barnes (1990) showed, sometimes the lack of choices and disempowerment of low status support workers mirrors the situation of their clients. Research by Ruth Marquis and Robert Jackson (2000) highlights the variable relationships which occur in living environment services for disabled people. Job descriptions stress tasks, not promoting autonomy or providing supportive relationships. Disabled people were clear that they wanted someone to share their life with them, and to be more than a worker. While this occurred in some care relationships, others verged on abuse. But Stacey (2005) shows that while homecare workers often feel constrained by their roles, they also find rewards and pride in what has been conceptualised as dirty and low-status work: her respondents sought emotional connections with clients and imported value and dignity into homecare.

The increasingly important role of non-disabled people committed to the empow-erment and inclusion of disabled people seems not to have received the attention it deserves. This constituency includes advocates and supporters of people with learning difficulties, those who are paid as personal assistants for disabled individ-uals, and perhaps also those who act as sign language interpreters or facilitate communication and inclusion in other ways. There are several important differences between what I will call support workers and traditional carers. The support service is typically paid, not voluntary; it is intermittent rather than continual; and the worker has usually made an active choice to engage in the work, often because of a political or ethical commitment to inclusion and empowerment. There are several important points arising from the role of support workers.

First, non-disabled people who work as advocates, personal assistants and interpreters are absolutely vital to the inclusion and independence of disabled people: without them, the voices and choices of people with learning difficulties would not be heard; physically dependent people would not be able to work or live independently; and Deaf people would find it much harder to negotiate the wider world.

Second, Dan Goodley argues that the role of non-disabled advocates for people with learning difficulties blurs the traditional disability rights distinction between organisations of disabled people and organisations for disabled people. 'Speaking out' and advocacy organisations are mainly staffed and run by non-disabled people, but for the benefit of people with learning difficulties. Jenny Walmsley highlighted this role of non-disabled supporters and researchers, suggesting that the 'normalisation philosophy gives non-disabled people a central and unassailable position' (Walmsley 2001: 194). Further, Goodley suggests that 'it is not professional involvement per se that limits or enables self-advocacy but the nature of interventions made by supporters in groups' (Goodley, 2001: 123). Allies, advocates, assistants and interpreters seem to lose their status as non-disabled people, enjoying the temporary privilege of membership of the disabled world.

Third, there has been very little attention to the motivations, views and experiences of these non-disabled support workers. In particular, the literature on independent living has failed adequately to include the perspectives of personal assistants. There has been such a strong focus on the need for choices, power and control being held by disabled people that there has been a neglect of the rights of their employees. Feminists have asked whether there is a danger of the emergence of a new servant class, comprising workers who are disproportionately female, usually from an unskilled or migrant workforce, rarely unionised, and likely to have poorer terms and conditions than the care workers traditionally employed by local authorities.

Drawing these themes together, I suggest that appreciation, respect and value needs to be accorded to those non-disabled people whose work is vital for the empowerment and independence of many disabled people:

> Unless personal assistance schemes can truly be a win–win situation for both employer (consumer) and employee (assistant), it will always be a 'nice idea', but one which is unstable in quality due to lack of incentive needed by those who probably would be proficient at peforming PAS but who need, as in any employment context, attractive wages, benefits and some type of opportunity for personal and professional advancement.
>
> (Marfisi, 2002: 28)

Understanding the situation of support workers, and what motivates them, is important to ensure that the supply of willing allies continues. For example, availability of direct payments is not sufficient, if disabled people persistently face problems in recruiting and retaining personal assistants.

This also points to possible future tensions, chiefly in the personal assistants/user relationship. The historical trajectory of most professions is towards improving status, knowledge and credentials, levering improved pay and conditions. If the different support worker roles become more formalised, and if there are problems with supply of suitable staff, there may be upward pressure on wages, and increasing conflicts for control between disabled people and the staff on whom they rely. Two factors suggest this may be unlikely: the political and ethical motivations of many workers, and the continuing supply of unskilled labour requiring flexible work opportunities.

## Researchers

Rejection of non-disabled researchers occurred at the beginnings of the British disability movement: E.J. Miller and E.V. Gwynne's research with residents of the Le Court Cheshire home was criticised as oppressive and demeaning. Ever since, there has been a suspicion of non-disabled researchers, who have been seen as parasitic on the lives of disabled people (Branfield, 1998). The goal of emancipatory research (Oliver, 1992a; Mercer, 2002) does not reject the role of non-disabled researchers, but does suggest that researchers need to follow the research agenda set by disabled people, and that accountability to organisations controlled by disabled people is very important. There have been considerable efforts to support disabled people and their organisations to become researchers and to manage research.

Just because someone is disabled does not mean they have an automatic insight into the lives of other disabled people. One person's experience may not be typical, and may actively mislead them as to the nature of disability. Because impairments are so diverse, someone with one impairment may have no more insight into the experience of another impairment than a person without any impairment. For example, most people researching with people with learning difficulties are non-disabled, but someone like Jan Walmsley or Dan Goodley has far more understanding of the situation of people with learning difficulties than a disabled academic such as myself. The idea that having an impairment is vital to understanding impairment is dangerously essentialist. The skills and knowledge of an experienced and sensitive researcher, disabled or non-disabled, are required to develop an appropriate account. Non-disabled researchers may be able to connect their own experiences of disempowerment or marginalisation – for example as women – to attain insight into the barriers experienced by disabled people (Duckett, 1998).

For example, Rannveig Traustadóttir (2001) offers a characteristically nuanced and reflexive account of her research with disabled people and other groups who are excluded and 'othered'. Dan Goodley and Michele Moore (2000) show how researchers can help facilitate the voices of people with learning difficulties and become engaged in political struggles, although they also record how academics are caught between the demands of university performance criteria, and their commitment to promoting the interests of disabled people:

> Our position as researchers who wish to be disabled people's allies, but who are situated within a context which requires us to contribute to the building up of a respectable discipline, presents real difficulties. We may wish to advance understanding of disability politics, but we are obliged to also maintain a definite position in the academy.
>
> (Goodley and Moore, 2000: 875)

Moreover, non-disabled people, as suggested previously, do have experiences of disability through their families. Dona Avery, quoted earlier, is a non-disabled parent of a disabled person. It is interesting to note that many non-disabled researchers active in disability studies are themselves first degree relatives of disabled people. As well as Avery, other parents of disabled people include Dora Barnason, Michael Berube, Eva Feder Kittay, Lars Grue; non-disabled children of disabled people include Lennard Davis and Rannveig Traustadóttir; and siblings include Eda Topliss. Each of these individuals will have experienced both 'courtesy stigma', but also the environmental and economic barriers placed on companions, carers and dependents of disabled people. Without the research contribution of the individuals named, and dozens of others including but not limited to Gary Albrecht, Len Barton, Mike Bury, Leanne Dowse, Kristjana Kristiansen, Geof Mercer, Mark Priestley, Bob Sapey, Mårten Söder and Linda Ward, the field of disability studies would never have developed to the status it currently enjoys.

## Conclusion

In this chapter I have tried to show that non-disabled people also have a stake in disability. In many different roles and relationships, impairment/disability issues touch their lives, and they have a role to play in supporting and enabling disabled people. People who have disabled family members, or people who devote their working lives to helping, researching or otherwise supporting disabled people have an interest in the social situation of disabled people, and in their improved quality of life.

Most disabled people have experienced negative treatment from non-disabled people. Lois Keith (1996) has written eloquently of the impact of unwanted attention or hostility:

> Disabled people have to work continually against destructive forces which see us as powerless, passive and unattractive. It seems that no matter how cheerfully and positively we attempt to go out into the world, we are bound

to be confronted by someone whose response to our lack of ordinariness, our difference from the norm leaves us feeling powerless and angry.

(Keith, 1996: 70)

Those who look different often face stares and mockery. Those who are vulnerable sometimes experience violence, abuse and hate crime. Naming and challenging this negative treatment has been an important step for the disability rights community. Yet these poor and sometimes dreadful experiences should not cause disabled people to assume that all non-disabled people will be rejecting or oppressive. I am convinced that many non-disabled people, most of the time, are accepting and supporting of disabled people. Where they fail adequately to respond, the problem is as likely to be ignorance and even fear as active hostility.

Disability activists and academics have a tendency to deny the possibility of non-disabled people taking a non-oppressive approach to disabled people. In an article in *Coalition* magazine, Alan Holdsworth (1993) divided the non-disabled world into three groups: professional oppressors, liberal oppressors and allies. For him, non-disabled people are the enemy: 'not only are they not our allies, but, in fact, are the beast itself' (1993: 4). Holdsworth's conception of what it takes to be an ally seems appropriate: 'An ally has to find ways of using all their skills, knowledge and abilities without taking over and without taking power away from disabled people' (1993: 5). Yet his polemic sees professionals and charity workers as self-interested, supporters of cuts in services, controlling their staff 'by a system of fear, cuts reorganisation and petty self interest' (1993: 7). Meanwhile 'liberal oppressors' mistakenly think they are on the side of the disability movement, rely on a charitable rather than a political response, support institutionalisation and refuse to allow disabled people to speak for themselves. Social research by Karin Barron (2001) deconstructs such crude polarities, showing that neither professionals nor parents are a homogenous group: some support the autonomy of disabled people, others exercise control, some try to protect, others act as advocates.

The polemical and separatist activist style, epitomised by Holdsworth's article, has poisoned relations between the disability movement and the professions and organisations which work in the disability field. In this chapter, I have tried to argue that the way forward lies in partnership and alliance between disabled people and non-disabled people and their organisations. Non-disabled people also have a stake in solving the disabilty problem. Professionals, carers and other helpers are more often motivated by an aspiration to help disabled people, than to oppress them. Those who want an easy working life which is well remunerated would be ill-advised to choose to work in the disability field, which has historically been of low status and pay. Most individual disabled people enjoy many good relationships with non-disabled people, as family members, workers, advocates and supporters. Yet collectively, the disability rights movement has chosen to ignore the positive aspects, and to highlight only the experiences of exclusion and oppression. A more realistic appraisal of the role of non-disabled people, recognising the way that their lives are often affected by disability, is long overdue.

# Chapter 13

# Concluding thoughts

In this book, I have re-examined some of the key principles of the British disability rights movement. I have questioned the intellectual and political basis for the social model of disability and the personal assistance model of independent living. I have also questioned the rejection of cure, genetic screening, assisted suicide and charity. Throughout the book, I have suggested that academics, activists and policy-makers need to look again at cherished rhetoric and taken-for-granted assumptions.

However, I want to stress three points. First, I accept that social and environmental barriers constitute major problems for many disabled people, and that removing such obstacles is the main priority for disability politics. Second, I agree that disabled people should have choices over their lives, and should be supported to live in the community. Third, I have no doubt that the medicalisation of disability and the persistent assumption that disabled people are defined by their incapacity are cultural barriers to the emancipation of disabled people which must be challenged. I welcome the UK Government's report on *Improving the Life Chances of Disabled People* (Cabinet Office, 2005), although I hope the focus on barriers and independent living does not obscure the needs of the most impaired disabled people.

I believe my account of disability suggests a practical research agenda. Disability studies should work to provide rich empirical studies, both quantitative and qualitative, of how disabled people experience barriers, and how they experience their impairments. In particular, the differences between disabled people are as important as the similarities: for example, examination of the role of class is paradoxically absent, even from materialist disability studies. Rather than being restricted by social model orthodoxy, disability studies should be pluralist, valuing analytical rigour and open debate. Disability researchers should look outwards and engage with medical sociology, bioethics and other areas of academia.

This book also highlights ways forward for emancipatory strategies. Disability movements should be cautious about assuming that either disability identity or disability rights are robust foundations for emancipation. Recognition that the majority of people with impairments have no desire to identify as disabled is overdue. So too is the appreciation that rights alone will not solve all disability problems (Young and Quibell, 2000; Barron, 2001): social justice may ultimately be the preferable goal. Disability groups should seek coalition with other parallel communities, particularly older people. It would be wrong to neglect either prevention of impairment or attention to the medical needs of disabled people. Finally, neither rights nor justice render concepts such as charity and community redundant. Supporting positive social relationships between disabled and non-disabled people and recognising the beneficial roles of solidarity and mutuality are both vital to the flourishing of disabled people.

# Bibliography

Abberley, P. (1987) The concept of oppression and the development of a social theory of disability, *Disability, Handicap and Society*, 2, 1, 5–20.

Abberley, P. (1992) Counting us out: a discussion of the OPCS disability surveys, *Disability, Handicap and Society*, 7, 2, 139–155.

Abberley, P. (1996) Work, utopia and impairment, in L.Barton (ed.) *Disability and Society: emerging issues and insights*, Harlow: Longman.

Abberley, P. (1998) The spectre at the feast: disabled people and social theory, in T. Shakespeare (ed.) *The Disability Reader: social science perspectives*, London: Cassell.

Abberley, P. (2001) Work, disability and European social theory, in C. Barnes, M. Oliver and L. Barton (eds) *Disability Studies Today*, Cambridge: Polity.

Abbott, D. and Howarth, J. (2005) *Secret Love, Hidden Lives? Exploring issues for people with learning difficulties who are gay, lesbian or bisexual*, Bristol: The Policy Press.

Abraham, C. (1989) Supporting people with mental handicap in the community: a social psychological perspective, *Disability, Handicap and Society*, 4, 2, 121–130.

Aitchison, C. (2003) From leisure and disability to disability leisure: developing data, definitions and discourses, *Disability and Society*, 18, 7, 955–969.

Albrecht, G.L. (ed.) (1976) *The Sociology of Physical Disability and Rehabilitation*, Pittsburgh, PA: University of Pittsburgh Press.

Albrecht, G.L. (ed.) (1981) *Cross National Rehabilitation Policies: a sociological perspective*, London: Sage.

Albrecht, G.L. (1992) *The Disability Business: rehabilitation in America*, London: Sage.

Albrecht, G.L. and Devlieger, P.J. (1999) The disability paradox: high quality of life against all odds, *Social Science and Medicine*, 48, 977–988.

Alderson, P. (1993) *Children's Consent to Surgery*, Buckingham: Open University Press.

Alderson, P. (2001) Down's syndrome: cost, quality and value of life, *Social Science and Medicine*, 53, 627–638.

Allison, R. (2003) Does a cleft palate justify an abortion? Curate wins right to challenge doctors, *Guardian*, 2 December.

Amundsen, R. (1992) Disability, handicap and the environment, *Journal of Social Philosophy*, 23, 1, 105–118.

Anderson, E. (1999) What is the point of equality? *Ethics*, 109, 287–337.

Andrews, J. (2005) Wheeling uphill? Reflections of practical and methodological difficulties encountered in researching the experiences of disabled volunteers, *Disability and Society*, 20, 2, 201–212.

Anspach, R.R. (1979) From stigma to identity politics, *Social Science and Medicine*, 134, 755–763.

Asch, A. (2000) Why I haven't changed my mind about prenatal diagnosis: reflections and refinements, in E. Parens and A. Asch (eds) *Prenatal Testing and Disability Rights*, Washington, DC: Georgetown University Press.

Asch, A. (2001) Disability, bioethics and human rights, in G.L. Albrecht, K.D. Seelman and M. Bury (eds) *Handbook of Disability Studies*, Thousand Oaks, CA: Sage.

Asch, A. and Geller, G. (1996) Feminism, bioethics, and genetics, in S.M. Wolf (ed.) *Feminism and Bioethics: Beyond reproduction*, New York: Oxford University Press.

Askheim, O.P. (2003) Personal assistance for people with intellectual impairments: experiences and dilemmas, *Disability and Society*, 18, 3, 325–340.

Askheim, O.P. (2005) Personal assistance – direct payments or alternative public service: Does it matter for the promotion of user control? *Disability and Society*, 20, 3, 247–260.

Atkin, K. and Hussain, Y. (2003) Disability and ethnicity: how young Asian disabled people make sense of their lives, in N. Watson and S. Riddell (eds) *Disability, Culture and Identity*, Harlow: Pearson Education.

Avery, D.M. (1999) Talking 'tragedy': identity issues in the parental story of disability, in M. Corker and S. French (eds) *Disability Discourse*, Buckingham: Open University Press.

Bailey, R. (1996) Prenatal testing and the prevention of impairment: a woman's right to choose? in J. Morris (ed.) *Encounters with Strangers: Feminism and Disability*, London: Women's Press.

Barnes, C. (1990) *The Cabbage Syndrome: the social construction of dependence*, Lewes: Falmer Press.

Barnes, C. (1991) *Disabled People in Britain and Discrimination*, London: Hurst and Co.

Barnes, C. (1995) Review of disability is not measles, edited by M. Rioux, *Disability and Society* 10, 3, 380.

Barnes, C. (1998a). Review of *The Rejected Body*, by Susan Wendell, *Disability and Society*, 13, 1, 145–147.

Barnes, C. (1998b) The social model of disability: a sociological phenomenon ignored by sociologists, in T. Shakespeare (ed.) *The Disability Reader*, London: Cassell.

Barnes, C. (1999) Disability studies: new or not-so-new directions, *Disability and Society*, 14, 4, 577–580.

Barnes, C. (2000) A working social model? Disability, work and disability politics in the 21st century, *Critical Social Policy*, 20, 4, 441–457.

Barnes, C. and Mercer, G. (1996) *Exploring the Divide: Illness and disability*, Leeds: The Disability Press.

Barnes, C. and Mercer, G. (2003) *Disability*, Cambridge: Polity.

Barnes C., and Mercer, G. (eds) (2004) *Implementing the Social Model of Disability: theory and research*, Leeds: The Disability Press.

Barnes, C., Oliver, M. and Barton, L. (eds) (2002) *Disability Studies Today*, Cambridge: Polity.

Barr, O., McConkey, R. and McConagahie, J. (2003) Views of people with learning difficulties about current and future accommodation: the use of focus groups to promote discussion, *Disability and Society*, 18, 5, 577–597.

Barron, K. (2001) Autonomy in everyday life, for whom? *Disability and Society*, 16, 3, 431–447.

Batavia, A.I. (1997) Disability and physician assisted suicide, *New England Journal of Medicine*, 336, 1671–1673.

Bates, P. and Davis, F.A. (2004) Social capital, social inclusion and services for people with learning disabilities, *Disability and Society*, 19, 3, 195–207.

Bauman, Z. (1992) *Mortality, Immortality and Other Life Strategies*, Cambridge: Polity.

Bauman, Z. (1993) *Postmodern Ethics*, Oxford: Blackwell.

Bauman, Z. (1998) On post-modern uses of sex, *Theory, Culture and Society*, 15, 3–4, 19–33.

BBC News website (2003) Euthanasia fears for disabled, 20 January. Online. Available HTTP: <http://news.bbc.co.uk/1/hi/health/2668253.stm> (accessed 24 January 2003).

Beardshaw, V. (1989) Conductive education: a rejoinder, *Disability, Handicap and Society*, 4, 3, 297–299.

Beck-Gernsheim, E. (1990) Changing duties of parents: from education to bio-engineering? *International Social Science Journal*, 42, 451.

Benjamin, A. (2004) Going undercover, *Guardian*, 14 April.

Beresford, P. and Wallcraft, J. (1997) Psychiatric system survivors and emancipatory research: issues, overlaps and differences, in C. Barnes and G. Mercer (eds) *Doing Disability Research*, Leeds: The Disability Press.

Beresford, P. and Wilson, A. (2002) Genes spell danger: mental health service users/ survivors, bioethics and control, *Disability and Society*, 17, 5, 541–553.

Berlin, I. (2000) Three Critics of the Enlightenment: Vico, Hamann, Herder, ed. Henry Hardy, London: Pimlico.

Bickenbach, J.E. (1993) *Physical Disability and Social Policy*, Toronto: University of Toronto Press.

Bickenbach, J. (1998) Disability and life-ending decisions, in M.P. Battin, R. Rhodes and A. Silvers (eds) *Physician Assisted Suicide: expanding the debate*, New York: Routledge.

Bickenbach, J.E., Chatterji, S., Badley, E.M. and Ustun, T.B. (1999) Models of disablement, universalism and the international classification of impairments, disabilities and handicaps, *Social Science and Medicine*, 48, 1173–1187.

Bjarnason, D. (2002) New voices in Iceland. Parents and adult children: juggling supports and choices in time and space, *Disability and Society*, 17, 3, 307–326.

Blaxter, M. (1976) *The Meaning of Disability*, London: Heinemann.

Bogdan, R. and Biklen D. (1993) Handicapism, in M. Nagler (ed.) *Text and Readings on Disability*, Palo Alto, CA: Health Markets Research.

Bornman, J. (2004) The World Health Organization's terminology and classification: application to severe disability, *Disability and Rehabilitation*, 26, 3, 182–188.

Bowe, F. (1978) *Handicapping America*, New York: Harper and Row.

Branfield, F. (1998) What are you doing here? 'Non-disabled' people and the disability movement: a response to Robert F. Drake, *Disability and Society*, 13, 1, 143–144.

Branfield, F. (1999) The disability movement: a movement of disabled people – a response to Paul S. Duckett, *Disability and Society*, 13, 3, 399–403.

Brechin, A. (1998) What makes for good care? in A. Brechin, J. Walmsley, J. Kalz and S. Peace (eds) *Care Matters: concepts, practice and research in health and social care*, London: Sage.

Brechin, A., Liddiard, P. and Swain, J. (eds) (1981) *Handicap in a Social World*, Sevenoaks: Hodder and Stoughton.

Brechin, A., Walmsley, J., Kalz, J. and Peace, S. (1998) *Care Matters: concepts, practice and research in health and social care*, London: Sage.

Brett, J. (2002) The experience of disability from the perspective of parents of children with profound impairment: is it time for an alternative model of disability? *Disability and Society*, 17, 7, 825–843.

Brisenden, S. (1989) Young, gifted and disabled: entering the employment market, *Disability, Handicap and Society*, 4, 3, 217–220.

British Council of Disabled People (n.d.) The social model of disability and emancipatory disability research – briefing document. Online. Available HTTP: <http://www.bcodp.org.uk/about/research.shtml> (accessed 23 March 2004).

Broberg, G. and Roll-Hansen, N. (eds) (1996) *Eugenics and the Welfare State: sterilization policies in Denmark, Sweden, Norway and Finland*, East Lansing, MI: Michigan State University Press.

Brouwer, W.B.F., Van Exel, N.J.A. and Stolk, E.A. (2005) Acceptability of less than perfect helath states, *Social Science and Medicine*, 60, 237–246.

Brown, N. (2003) Hope against hype – accountability in biopasts, presents and futures, *Science Studies*, 16, 2, 3–21.

Brown, N. and Michael, M.A. (2003) The sociology of expectations: retrospecting prospects and prospecting retrospects, *Technology Analysis and Strategic Management*, 15, 1, 3–19.

Brown, P. (1995) Naming and framing: the social construction of diagnosis and illness, *Journal of Health and Social Behaviour* (extra issue), 34–52.

Brunner, E. (1997) Socioeconomic determinants of health: stress and the biology of inequality, *British Medical Journal*, 314, 1472–1476.

Buchanan, A. (1996) Choosing who will be disabled: genetic intervention and the morality of inclusion, *Social Philosophy and Policy*, 13, 2, 18–46.

Buchanan, A., Brock, D.W., Daniels, N. and Wikler, D. (2000) *From Chance to Choice: genetics and justice*, Cambridge: Cambridge University Press.

Burleigh, M. (1994) *Death and Deliverance: 'Euthanasia' in Germany 1900–1945*, Cambridge: Cambridge University Press.

Burleigh, M. (1998) *Ethics and Extermination: reflections on Nazi genocide*, Cambridge: Cambridge University Press.

Burrows, G. (2003) A piece of the action, *Guardian*, 5 November.

Bury, M. (1996) Defining and researching disability: challenges and responses, in C. Barnes and G. Mercer (eds) *Exploring the Divide: chronic illness and disability*, Leeds: The Disability Press.

Bury, M. (1997) *Health and Illness in a Changing Society*, London: Routledge.

Bury, M. (2000) A comment on the ICIDH2, *Disability and Society*, 15, 7, 1073–1077.

Butler, J. (1990) *Gender Trouble: feminism and the subversion of identity*, New York: Routledge.

Bytheway, B. and Johnson, J. (1998) The social construction of 'carers', in A. Symonds and A. Kelly (eds) *The Social Construction of Community Care*, Basingstoke: Macmillan.

Cabinet Office (2005) *Improving the Life Chances of Disabled People*, London: The Stationery Office.

Callahan, D. (2003) Principlism and communitarianism, *Journal of Medical Ethics*, 29, 287–291.

Campbell, J. (2003) Don't be fooled, we don't all want to kill ourselves. Online. Available HTTP: <http://www.bcodp.org.uk/about/campbell.shtml> (accessed 23 March 2004).

Campbell, J. and Oliver, M. (1996) *Disability Politics: understanding our past, changing our future*, London: Routledge.

Caplan, A.L., McGee, G. and Magnus, D. (1999) What is immoral about eugenics? *British Medical Journal*, 319, 1284.

Carmichael, A. and Brown, L. (2002) The future challenges for direct payments, *Disability and Society*, 17, 7, 797–808.

Carpenter, M. (1994) *Normality is Hard Work: trades unions and the politics of community care*, London: Lawrence and Wishart.

Carr, L. (2000) Enabling our destruction? *Coalition*, August, 29–36.

Carvel, J. (2004) Demonstrators rattle Scope, *Guardian*, 6 October.

Carvel, J (2005) Scope for improvement: disability charity shifts its policy towards integration, *Guardian*, 2 March.

Carver, V. and Rodda, M. (1978) *Disability and the Environment*, London: Elek Books.

Centre for Universal Design (1997) *The Principles of Universal Design*. Online. Available HTTP:<http://www.design.ncsu.edu/cud/univ_design/principles/udprinciples.htm> (accessed 24 August 2004).

Chadwick, A. (1996) Knowledge, power and the Disability Discrimination Bill, *Disability and Society*, 11, 1, 25–40.

Chappell, A. (1998) Still out in the cold: people with learning difficulties and the social model of disability, in T. Shakespeare (ed.) *The Disability Reader*, London: Cassell.

Chappell, A.L., Goodley, D. and Lawthom, R. (2001) Making connections: the relevance of the social model of disability for people with learning difficulties, *British Journal of Learning Disabilities*, 24, 45–50.

Charlton, J. (1998) *Nothing About Us Without Us: Disability, oppression and empowerment*, Berkeley: University of California Press.

Cherniack, E.P. (2002) Increasing use of DNR orders in the elderly worldwide: whose choice is it? *Journal of Medical Ethics*, 28, 303–307.

Clarke, C.L., Lhussier, M., Minto, C., Gibb, C.E. and Perini, T. (2005) Paradoxes, locations and the need for social coherence: a qualitative study of living with a learning difficulty, *Disability and Society*, 20, 4, 405–420.

Clear, M. (ed.) (2000) *Promises, Promise: disability and terms of inclusion*, Sydney: Federation Press.

Coles, J. (2001) The social model of disability: what does it mean for practice in services for people with learning difficulties? *Disability and Society*, 16, 4, 501–510.

Colver, A. (2005) A shared framework and language for childhood disability, *Developmental Medicine and Child Neurology*, 47, 780–784.

Conrad, P. and Schneider, J.W. (1992) *Deviance and Medicalization*, Philadelphia: Temple University Press.

Conrad, P. and Potter, D. (2004) Human growth hormone and the temptations of biomedical enhancement, *Sociology of Health and Illness*, 26, 2, 184–215.

Cooper, C. (1997) Can a fat woman call herself disabled? *Disability and Society*, 12, 1, 31–42.

Cooper, M. (1999) The Australian disability rights movement lives, *Disability and Society*, 14, 2, 217–226.

Corker, M. (1998) *Deaf and Disabled or Deafness Disabled*, Buckingham: Open University Press.

Corker, M. (1999) Conflations, differences and foundations: the limits to 'accurate' theoretical representation of disabled people's experience? *Disability and Society*, 14, 5, 627–642.

Corker, M. and French, S. (eds) (1999) *Disability Discourse*, Buckingham: Open University Press.

Crewe, N.M. and Zola, I.K. (eds) (1983) *Independent Living for Physically Disabled People*, San Francisco, CA: Jossey-Bass Publishers.

Crow, L. (1991) Rippling raspberries: disabled women and sexuality, unpublished M.Sc. dissertation, South Bank Polytechnic.

Crow, L. (1992) Renewing the social model of disability, *Coalition*, July, 5–9.

Crow, L. (1996) Including all our lives, in J. Morris (ed.) *Encounters with Strangers: feminism and disability*, London: Women's Press.

Dalley, G. (1988) *Ideologies of Caring: rethinking community and collectivism*, London: Macmillan.

Danermark, B. and Gellerstedt, L.C. (2004) Social justice: redistribution and recognition – a non-reductionist perspective on disability, *Disability and Society*, 19, 4, 339–353.

Darke, P. (2004) Interview: beyond the U bend, *Disability Arts in London*, 182, 15–17.

Darling, R.B. (2003) Towards a model of changing disability identities: a proposed typology and research agenda, *Disability and Society*, 18, 7, 881–895.

Davis, A. (2004) A disabled person's perspective on euthanasia, paper presented at UK Forum on Healthcare Law and Ethics, University of Newcastle.

Davis, C. (1998) Caregiving, carework and professional care, in A. Brechin, J. Walmsley, J. Katz and S. Peace (eds) *Care Matters: concepts, practice and research in health and social care*, London: Sage.

Davis, F. (1964) Deviance disavowal and the visibly handicapped, in H. Becker (ed.) *The Other Side*, New York: Free Press.

Davis, K. (1993) On the movement, in J. Swain *et al.* (eds) *Disabling Barriers, Enabling Environments*, London: Sage.

Davis, L.J. (1995) *Enforcing Normalcy: disability, deafness and the body*, London: Verso.

Davis, L.J. (2002) *Bending over Backwards: disability, dismodernism and other difficult positions*, New York: New York University Press.

Deal, M. (2003) Disabled people's attitudes towards other impairment groups: a hierachy of impairment, *Disability and Society*, 18, 7, 897–910.

Deeley, S. (2002) Professional ideology and learning disability: an analysis of internal conflict, *Disability and Society*, 17, 1, 19–33.

DeJong, G. (1983) Defining and implementing the Independent Living concept, in N. Crewe and I. Zola (eds) *Independent Living for Physically Disabled People*, London: Jossey Bass.

Department for Work and Pensions (2003) *Disabled for Life?* London: DWP.

Department of Health (2001) *Valuing People*, London: DoH.

Department of Health Community Care Statistics (2003–04) *Referrals, Assessments and Packages of Care For Adults, England: National Summary*. Online. Available HTTP: <http://www.publications.doh.gov.uk/rap/rap-report2003-4.doc> (accessed 17 June 2005).

Despouy, L. (1993) *Human Rights and Disability*, New York: United Nations Economic and Social Council.

De Swaan, A. (1990) *The Management of Normality: critical essays in health and welfare*, London: Routledge.

De Wolfe, P. (2002) Private tragedy in social context? Reflections on disability, illness and suffering, *Disability and Society*, 17, 3, 255–267.

Diem, S.J., Lantos, J.D. and Tulsky, J.A. (1996) Cardiopulmonary resuscitation on television: Miracles and misinformation, *New England Journal of Medicine*, 13, 334, 24, 1578–1582.

Disability Awareness in Action (1997) *Life, Death and Rights: Bioethics and Disabled People*, special supplement, Disability Awareness in Action, London.

Disability Awareness in Action (2003) UK hospital's new policy puts pressure on people to refuse treatment, *Disability Tribune*, March, 1.

Disability Awareness in Action (n.d.a) *Disability Awareness in Action* newsletter. Online. Available HTTP: <http://www.daa.org.uk/biotech_special.htm>

Disability Awareness in Action (n.d.b) Social model or unsociable model? Online. Available HTTP: <www.daa.org.uk/social_model.html> (accessed 26 April 2004).

DisAbility Services (n.d.) Community inclusion – enhancing friendship networks among people with a cognitive impairment, Victorian Government Department of Human Services. Online. Available HTTP: <http://www.dhs.vic.gov.au/disability> (accessed July 2005).

Disabled People's International (1982) Proceedings of the First World Congress, Singapore, Singapore: Disabled People's International.

Dowling, M. and Dolan, L. (2001) Families of children with disabilities – inequalities and the social model, *Disability and Society*, 16, 1, 21–36.

Doyle, B. (1996) *Disability Discrimination: The new law*, London: Jordans.

Drake, R.F. (1996) A critique of the role of the traditional charities, in L. Barton (ed.) *Disability and Society: emerging issues and insights*, Harlow: Longman.

Dreidger, D. (1989) *The Last Civil Rights Movement*, London: Hurst.

Duckett, P.S. (1998) What are you doing here? 'Non disabled people' and the disability movement: a response to Fran Branfield, *Disability and Society*, 13, 4, 625–628.

Duffield, V.L. (2001) Friendship and autistic spectrum disorders: a practical programme, *International Journal of Practical Approaches to Disability*, 25, 1, 43.

Dworkin, R.M. (1984) *Life's Dominion: an argument about abortion, euthanasia and individual freedom*, New York: Vintage Books.

Eagle, M., Baudouin, S., Chandler, C., Giddings, D., Bullock, R. and Bushby, K. (2002) Survival in Duchene muscular dystrophy: improvements in life expectancy since 1967 and the impact of home nocturnal ventilation, *Neuromuscular Disorders*, 12, 10, 926–929.

Earle, S. (1999) Facilitated sex and the concept of sexual need: disabled students and their personal assistants, *Disability and Society*, 14, 3, 309–324.

Edgerton, R. (1984) *The Cloak of Competence: stigma in the lives of the mentally retarded*, Berkeley: University of California Press.

Edwards, S.D. (2004) Disability, identity and the 'expressivist objection', *Journal of Medical Ethics*, 30, 418–420.

Edwards, S.D. (2005) *Disability: definitions, value and identity*, Abingdon: Radcliffe.

Eleweke, C.J. (1999) The need for mandatory legislation to enhance services to people with disabilities in Nigeria, *Disability and Society*, 14, 2, 227–238.

Elliot, C. (1999) Pursued by happiness and beaten senseless: Prozac and the American Dream, *Hastings Center Report*, 30, 2, 7–12.

Emerson, E. and McVilly, K. (2004) Friendship activities of adults with intellectual disabilities in supported accommodation in Northern England, *Journal of Applied Research in Intellectual Disabilities*, 17, 191–197.

Epstein, R. (2005) The right to die: the assisted dying for the terminally ill bill, *Legal Executive Journal*, September, 14–16.

Fausto-Sterling, A. (2003) The problem with sex/gender and nature/nurture, in S.J. Williams, L. Birke and G.A. Bendelow (eds) *Debating Biology: sociological reflections on health, medicine and society*, London: Routledge.

Ferguson, I. (2003) Challenging a 'spoiled identity': mental health service users, recognition and redistribution, in N. Watson and S. Riddell (eds) *Disability, Culture and Identity*, Harlow: Pearson Education.

Finch, J. (1984) Community care: developing non-sexist alternatives, *Critical Social Policy*, 9, 6–18.

Findlay, B. (1999) Disability rights and culture under attack, *Disability Arts in London*, 149 (July), 6–7.

Finger, A. (1992) Forbidden fruit, *New Internationalist*, 233, 8–10.

Finkelstein, V. (1980) *Attitudes and Disabled People*, New York: World Rehabilitation Fund.

Finkelstein, V. (1981) To deny or not to deny disability, in A. Brechin, P. Liddiard and J. Swain (eds) *Handicap in a Social World*, Sevenoaks: Hodder and Stoughton.

Finkelstein, V. (2001) *A Personal Journey into Disability Politics*, Leeds: University of Leeds, Centre for Disability Studies.

Finkelstein, V., French, S. and Oliver, M. (eds) (1993) *Disabling Barriers, Enabling Environments*, London: OUP/Sage.

Finlay, I.G., Wheatley, V.J. and Izdebski, C. (2005) The House of Lords Select Committee on the Assisted Dying for the Terminally Ill Bill: implications for specialist palliative care, *Palliative Medicine*, 19, 444–453.

Finlay, M. and Lyons, E. (1998) Social identity and people with learning difficulties: implications for self-advocacy groups, *Disability and Society*, 13, 1, 37–52.

Fisher, B. and Galler, R. (1988) Friendship and fairness: how disability affects friendship between women, in M. Fine and A. Asch (eds) *Women with Disabilities: essays in psychology, culture and politics*, Philadelphia: Temple University Press.

Fitzgerald, J. (1999) Bioethics, disability and death: uncovering cultural bias in the euthanasia debate, in M. Jones and L. Basser Marks (eds) *Disability, Divers-Ability and Legal Change*, The Hague: Martinus Nijhoff Publishers.

Fletcher, A. (1999) *Genes are us? Attitudes to genetics and disability*, London: RADAR.

Fletcher, A. (2006) What's in a name? *Disability Now*, January, 21.

Flory, J.H. and Kitcher, P. (2004) Global health and the scientific research agenda, *Philosophy and Public Affairs*, 32, 1, 36–65.

Foucault, M. (1989) *The History of Sexuality, Volume 1*, Harmondsworth: Penguin.

Foucault, M. (1990) *Politics, Philosophy, Culture*, London: Routledge.

Fox, H.M. and Kim, K. (2004) Understanding emerging disabilities, *Disability and Society*, 19, 4, 323–337.

Frank, E., Anderson, C. and Rubinstein, D. (1978) Frequency of sexual dysfunction in 'normal' couples, *New England Journal of Medicine*, 299, 111–115.

Franklin, S. (2003) Ethical biocapital: new strategies of cell culture, in S. Franklin and M. Lock (eds) *Rethinking Life and Death: towards an anthropology of the biosciences*, Santa Fe, NM: School of American Research Press.

Fraser, N. (1989) *Unruly Practices: power, discourse and gender in contemporary social theory*, Minneapolis, MN: University of Minnesota Press.

Fraser, N. (1995) From redistribution to recognition, *New Left Review*, 212, 68–92.

Fraser, N. (2000) Rethnking recognition, *New Left Review*, 3, 107–120.

Fraser, N. and Nicholson, L. (1990) Social criticism without philosophy: an encounter between feminism and postmodernism, in L. Nicholson (ed.) *Feminism/Postmodernism*, London: Routledge.

Fraser, W.I. (1992) The professions, knowledge and practice, in S.R. Barron and J.D. Haldane (eds) *Community, Normality and Difference*, Aberdeen: Aberdeen University Press.

Freidson, E. (1970) *Profession of Medicine: a study of the sociology of applied knowledge*, New York: Harper and Row.

Freire, P. (1972) *The Pedagogy of the Oppressed*, Harmondsworth: Penguin.

French, S. (1988) Experiences of disabled health and caring professionals, *Sociology of Health and Illness*, 10, 2, 170–188.

French, S. (1993) Disability, impairment or something in between, in J. Swain, S. French, C. Barnes and C. Thomas (eds) *Disabling Barriers, Enabling Environments*, London: Sage.

Freund, P. (1988) Bringing society into the body: understanding socialized human nature, *Theory and Society*, 17, 839–864.

Freund, P. (2001) Bodies, disability and spaces: the social model and disabling spatial organisations, *Disability and Society*, 16, 5, 689–706.

Friedman, M. (1993) Beyond caring: the de-moralization of gender, in M.J. Larrabee (ed.) *An Ethic of Care: feminist and interdisciplinary perspectives*, New York: Routledge.

Fuss, D. (1989) *Essentially Speaking: feminism, nature and difference*, New York: Routledge.

Gabel, S. and Peters, S. (2004) Presage of a paradigm shift? Beyond the social model of disability toward resistance theories of disability, *Disability and Society*, 19, 6, 585–600.

Gaita, R. (2002) *The Philosopher's Dog*, Melbourne: Text Publishing.

Gallagher, H. (1995) *By Trust Betrayed: patients, physicians and the licence to kill in the Third Reich*, New York: Vandemere Press.

Galvin, R. (2003) The paradox of disability culture: the need to combine versus the imperative to let go, *Disability and Society*, 18, 5, 675–690.

Ganchoff, C. (2004) Regenerating movements: embryonic stem cells and the politics of potentiality, *Sociology of Health and Illness*, 26, 6, 757–774.

Gardiner, P. (2003) A virtue ethics approach to moral dilemmas in medicine, *Journal of Medical Ethics*, 29, 297–302.

Gazelle, G. (1998) The slow code – should anyone rush to its defense? *New England Journal of Medicine*, 338, 467–469.

Gill, C.J. (1992) Suicide intervention for people with disabilities: a lesson in inequality, *Issues in Law and Medicine*, 8, 1, 37–53.

Gill, C.J. (1994) Questioning continuum, in B. Shaw (ed.) *The Ragged Edge*, Louisville, KY: Avocado Press.

Gill, C.J. (2000) Health professionals, disability and assisted suicide: an examination of relevant empirical evidence and reply to Batavia, *Psychology, Public Policy and Law*, 6, 2, 526–545.

Gilligan, C. (1983) *In a Different Voice: psychological theory and women's development*, Cambridge, MA: Harvard University Press.

Gillman, M., Heyman, B. and Swain, J. (2000) What's in a name? The implications of diagnosis for people with learning difficulties and their family carers, *Disability and Society*, 15, 3, 389–409.

Gillon, R (2001) Is there a 'new ethics of abortion'? *Journal of Medical Ethics*, 27 supplement II, ii5–ii9.

Gilson, S.F., Tusler, A. and Gill, C. (1997) Ethnographic research in disability identity, self-determination and community, *Journal of Vocational Rehabilitation*, 9, 7–17.

Girlin, T. (1990) From universality to difference, in C. Calhoun (ed.) *Social Theory and the Politics of Identity*, Cambridge, MA: Blackwell.

Glendinning, C., Rummery, K., Halliwell, S., Jacobs, S. and Tyrer, J. (2000) *Buying Independence: using direct payments to purchase integrated health and social services*, Bristol: The Policy Press.

Glover, J. (1977) *Causing Death and Saving Lives*, Harmondsworth: Penguin.

Goffman, E. (1968a) *Stigma: notes on the management of spoiled identity*, Harmondsworth: Penguin.

Goffman, E. (1968b) *Asylums: essays on the social situation of mental patients and other inmates*, Harmondsworth: Penguin.

Goggin, G. and Newell, C. (2004) Uniting the nation? Disability, stem cells and the Australian media, *Disability and Society*, 19, 1, 47–60.

Goggin, G. and Newell, C. (2005) *Disability in Australia: exposing a social apartheid*, Sydney: UNSW Press.

Gold, D. (1999) Friendship, leisure and support: the purposes of 'circles of friends' of young people, *Journal of Leisurability*, 26, 3, 1–13.

Gooding, C. (2000) Disability Discrimination Act: from statute to practice, *Critical Social Policy*, 20, 4, 533–549.

Goodley, D. and Moore, M. (2000) Doing disability research: activist lives and the academy, *Disability and Society*, 15, 6, 861–882.

Goodley, D. (2001) 'Learning difficulties', the social model of disability and impairment: challenging epistemologies, *Disability and Society*, 16, 2, 207–231.

Goodley, D. (2003) Against a politics of victimisation: disability culture and self-advocates with learning difficulties, in N. Watson and S. Riddell (eds) *Disability, Culture and Identity*, Harlow: Pearson Education.

Gordon, B.O. and Rosenblum, K.E. (2001) Bringing disability into the sociological frame: a comparison of disability with race, sex and sexual orientation statuses, *Disability and Society*, 16, 1, 5–19.

Gosling, V. and Cotterill, L. (2000) An employment project as a route to social inclusion for people with learning difficulties? *Disability and Society*, 15, 7, 1001–1018.

Graham, H. (1983) Caring: a labour of love, in J. Finch and D. Groves (eds) *A Labour of Love: women, work and caring*, London: Routledge & Kegan Paul.

Graham, H. (1991) The concept of caring in feminist research: the case of domestic service, *Sociology*, 25, 1, 61–78.

Grey-Thompson, T. (2005) Tactile paving and other bad inventions. Online. Available HTTP: <http://www.bbc.co.uk/ouch/columnists/tanni/130605_index.shtml> (accessed 1 August 2005).

Groce, N. (1985) *Everyone Here Spoke Sign Language: hereditary deafness on Martha's Vineyard*, Cambridge, MA: Harvard University Press.

Gustavsson, A. (2004) The role of theory in disability research: springboard or strait-jacket? *Scandinavian Journal of Disability Research*, 6, 1, 55–70.

Gustavsson, A., Sandvin, J., Traustadóttir R., Tøssebro J. (2005) *Resistance, Reflection and Change: Nordic disability research*, Lund: Studentlitteratur.

Hacking, I. (1986) Making up people, in T.C. Helier, M. Sosna and D.E. Wellbery, *Reconstructing Individualism*, Stanford: Stanford University Press.

Hacking, I. (2000) *The Social Construction of What?* Cambridge, MA: Harvard University Press.

Hahn, H. (1985) Towards a politics of disability: definitions, disciplines and policies, *Social Science Journal*, 22, 4, 87–105.

Hahn, H. (1986) Public support for rehabilitation programs: the analysis of US disability policy, *Disability, Handicap and Society*, 1, 121–138.

Hahn, H. (1988) The politics of physical differences: disability and discrimination, *Journal of Social Issues*, 44, 1, 39–47.

Hampton, S.J. (2005) Family eugenics, *Disability and Society*, 20, 5, 553–561.

Happé, F. (1994) *Autism: an introduction to psychological theory*, London: UCL Press.

Haraway, D. (1988) Situated knowledges: the science question in feminism and the privilege of partial perspective, *Feminist Studies*, 3, 575–599.

Harden, J. (2005) Parenting a young person with mental health problems: temporary disruption and reconstruction, *Sociology of Health and Illness*, 27, 3, 351–371.

Harris, J. (1985) *The Value of Life: an introduction to medical ethics*, London: Routledge Kegan Paul.

Harris, J. (1992) *Wonderwoman and Superman: the ethics of human biotechnology*, Oxford: Oxford University Press.

Harris, J. (1993) Is gene therapy a form of eugenics? *Bioethics*, 7, 178–187.

Harris, J. (2000) The welfare of the child, *Health Care Analysis*, 8, 1, 27–34.

Harris, J. (2001) One principle and three fallacies of disability studies, *Journal of Medical Ethics*, 27, 6, 383–388.

Harris, J. and Bamford, C. (2001) Services for Deaf and hard of hearing people, *Disability and Society*, 16, 7, 969–979.

Harris, M. and Rochester, C. (2001) *Voluntary Organisations and Social Policy in Britain: Perspectives on change and choice*, Basingstoke: Palgrave.

Hasler, F. (1993) Developments in the disabled people's movement, in J. Swain, S. French, C. Barnes and C. Thomas (eds) *Disabling Barriers – Enabling Environments*, London: Sage.

Hasler, F. (2003) Clarifying the evidence on direct payments into practice. Online. Available HTTP: <http://www.ncil.org.uk/evidence_paper.asp> (accessed 4 March 2004).

Hedlund, M. (2000) Disability as a phenomenon: a discourse of social and biological understandings, *Disability and Society*, 15, 5, 765–780.

Helgøy, I., Ravenberg, B. and Solvang, P. (2003) Service provision for an independent life, *Disability and Society*, 18, 4, 471–487.

Henderson, J. and Forbat, L. (2002) Relationship-based social policy: personal and policy constructions of 'care', *Critical Social Policy*, 72, 22, 4, 669–687.

Henley, C.A. (2001) Good intentions – unpredicatable consequences, *Disability and Society*, 16, 7, 933–947.

Henn, W. (2000) Consumerism in prenatal diagnosis: a challenge for ethical guidelines, *Journal of Medical Ethics*, 26, 444–446.

Hevey, D. (1992) *The Creatures Time Forgot: photography and disability imagery*, London: Routledge.

Hilberman, M., Kutner, J., Parsons, D. and Murphy D.J. (1997) Marginally effective medical care: ethical analysis of issues in cardiopulmonary resuscitation, *Journal of Medical Ethics*, 23, 361–7.

Hodge, N. (2005) Reflections on diagnosing autism spectrum disorders, *Disability and Society*, 20, 3, 345–349.

Holdsworth, A. (1993) Our allies within, *Coalition*, June, 4–10.

Honneth, A. (1995) *The Struggle for Recognition: the moral grammar of social conflicts*, Cambridge: Polity.

Hood-Williams, J. (1996). Goodbye to sex and gender, *Sociological Review*, 44, 1, 1–16.

Hughes, B., McKie, L., Hopkins, D. and Watson, N. (2005) Love's labour's lost? Feminism, the disabled people's movement and an ethic of care, *Sociology*, 39, 2, 259–275.

Hughes, B., Russell, R. and Paterson, K. (2005) Nothing to be had 'off the peg': consumption, identity and the immobilization of young disabled people, *Disability and Society*, 20, 1, 3–18.

Humphrey, J.C. (1999) Disabled people and the politics of difference, *Disability and Society*, 14, 173–188.

Humphrey, J.C. (2000) Researching disability politics, or, some problems with the social model in practice, *Disability and Society*, 15, 1, 63–85.

Hunt, P. (ed.) (1966) *Stigma*, London: Geoffrey Chapman Publishing.

Hurst, R. (1995) Choice and empowerment – lessons from Europe, *Disability and Society*, 10, 4, 529–534.

Hurst, R. (ed.) (1998) *Are Disabled People Included?* London: Disability Awareness in Action.

Hurst, R. (2000) To revise or not to revise, *Disability and Society*, 15, 7, 1083–1087.

Hurst, R. (n.d.) Assisted suicide and disabled people: a briefing paper. Online. Available HTTP: <http://wwww.daa.org.uk/assisted_suicide.htm> (accessed 26 April 2004).

Huurre, T.M. and Aro, H.M. (1998) Psychosocial development among adolescents with visual impairment, *European Child and Adolescent Psychiatry*, 7, 73–78.

Hyde, M. (1996) Fifty years of failure: employment services for disabled people in the UK, *Work, Employment and Society*, 12 , 3, 683–700.

Illich, I. (1977) *Limits to Medicine*, New York: Penguin.

Imrie, R. (2004) Demystifying disability: a review of the International Classification of Functioning, Disability and Health, *Sociology of Health and Illness*, 26, 3, 287–305.

Ineland, J. (2005) Logics and discourses in disability arts in Sweden: a neo-institutional perspective, *Disability and Society*, 20, 7, 749–762.

Jamieson, L. (1998) *Intimacy: personal relationships in modern society*, Cambridge: Polity.

Jay, N. (1981) Gender and dichotomy, *Feminist Studies*, 7, 38–56.

Juengst, E.T. (1998) What does enhancement mean? in E. Parens (ed.) *Enhancing Human Traits: social and ethical implications*, Washington, DC: Georgetown University Press.

Keith, L. (1996) Encounters with strangers, in J. Morris (ed.) *Encounters with Strangers: disability and feminism*, London: Women's Press.

Kelly, B (2005) 'Chocolate . . . makes you autism': impairment, disability and childhood identities, *Disability and Society*, 20, 3, 261–276.

Kelly, M.P. and Field, D. (1996) Medical sociology, chronic illness and the body, *Sociology of Health and Illness*, 18, 2, 241–257.

Kelly, M.P. and Field, D. (1994) Reflections on the rejection of the bio-medical model in sociological discourse, *Medical Sociology News*, 19, 34–37.

Kerr, A. and Shakespeare, T. (2002) *Genetic Politics: from eugenics to genome*, Cheltenham, New Clarion Press.

Kevles, D.J. (1985) *In the Name of Eugenics: genetics and the uses of human heredity*, New York: Knopf.

King, D.S. (1999) Preimplantation genetic diagnosis and the 'new' eugenics, *Journal of Medical Ethics*, 25, 2, 176–182.

Kitcher, P. (1997 ) *Lives to Come: the genetic revolution and human possibilities*, New York: Simon and Schuster.

Kittay, E.F. (1999) *Love's Labour: essays on women, equality and dependency*, New York: Routledge.

Kripke, S. (1980) *Naming and Necessity*, Oxford: Blackwell.

Kritzman, L.D. (ed.) (1990) *Michel Foucault: politics, philosophy, culture*, New York: Routledge.

Kuczewski, M.G. (2001) Disability: an agenda for bioethics, *American Journal of Bioethics*, 1, 3, 36–44.

Kuhn, T. (1970) *The Structure of Scientific Revolutions*, Chicago, IL: University of Chicago Press.

Kuhse, H. and Singer, P. (1985) *Should the Baby Live? The problem of handicapped infants*, Oxford: Oxford University Press.

Larrabee, M.J. (ed.) (1993) *An Ethic of Care: feminist and interdisciplinary perspectives*, New York: Routledge.

Laura, R.S. (ed.) (1980) *Problems of Handicap*, Melbourne: Macmillan.

Lee, P. (2002) Shooting for the moon: politics and disability at the beginning of the twenty-first century, in C. Barnes, M. Oliver and L. Barton (eds) *Disability Studies Today*, Cambridge: Polity.

Lee-Treweek, G. (1996) Emotion work in care assistant work, in V. James and J. Gabe (eds) *Health and the Sociology of the Emotions*, Oxford: Blackwell.

Leff, J. (2001) *The Unbalanced Mind*, London: Phoenix.

Leipoldt, E. (2005) Embryonic stem cell research: a sob story. Online. Available HTTP: <www.onlineopinion.com.au/print.asp?article=172> (accessed 10 October).

Lenney, M. and Sercombe, H. (2002) 'Did you see that guy in the wheelchair down the pub?' Interactions across difference in a public place, *Disability and Society*, 17, 1, 5–18.

Lester, H. and Tritter, J.Q. (2005) 'Listen to my madness': understanding the experiences of people with serious mental illness, *Sociology of Health and Illness*, 27, 5, 649–669.

Levy, N. (2002) Reconsidering cochlear implants: the lesson of Martha's Vineyard, *Bioethics*, 16, 2, 134–153.

Lifton, R.J. (1986) *The Nazi Doctors: medical killing and the psychology of genocide*, London: Macmillan.

Liggett, H. (1988) Stars are not born: an interpretative approach to the politics of disability, *Disability, Handicap and Society*, 3, 3, 263–276.

Linton, S. (1998) *Claiming Disability: knowledge and identity*, New York: New York University Press.

Lippman, A. (1994) Prenatal genetic testing and screening: constructing needs and reinforcing inequalities, in A. Clarke (ed.) *Genetic Counselling: practice and principles*, London: Routledge.

Lister, R. (1997) *Citizenship: feminist perspectives*, Basingstoke: Macmillan.

Littlewood, J. (2004) Looking back over 40 years and what the future holds: Joseph Levy Memorial Lecture and the Ettore Rossi Medal Lecture, 27th European Cystic Fibrosis Conference, Birmingham.

Llewellyn, A. and Hogan, K. (2000) The use and abuse of models of disability, *Disability and Society*, 15, 1, 157–165.

Lock, S., Jordan, L., Bryan, K. and Maxim, J. (2005) Work after stroke: focusing on barriers and enablers, *Disability and Society*, 20, 1, 33–47.

Locker, D. (1983) *Disability and Disadvantage*, London: Tavistock.

Longmore, P.K. (1997) Conspicuous contribution and American cultural dilemmas: telethon rituals of cleansing and renewal, in D.T. Mitchell and S.L. Synder (eds) *The Body and Physical Difference: discourses of disability*, Ann Arbor, MI: University of Michigan.

Longmore, P.K. (2002) *Why I Burned My Book and Other Essays on Disability*, Philadelphia: Temple University Press.

Lynch, K. and McLaughlin, E. (1995) Caring labour and love labour, in P. Clancy, S. Drudy, K. Lynch and L. O'Dowd (eds) *Irish Society: sociological perspecitves*, Dublin: Institute of Public Administration.

Macintyre, A. (1999) *Dependent Rational Animals: why human beings need the virtues*, London: Duckworth.

McLaughlin, E. and Glendinning, C. (1994) Paying for care in Europe: is there a feminist approach? in L. Hantrais and S. Mangan (eds) *Family Policy and the Welfare of Women*, Cross National Research Papers, London: ESRC.

Mclaughlin, J. (2003) Screening networks: shared agendas in feminist and disability movement challenges to antenatal screening and abortion, *Disability and Society*, 18, 3, 297–310.

Maclean, A. (1993) *The Elimination of Morality: reflections on utilitarianism and bioethics*, London: Routledge.

Madigan, R. and Milner, J. (1999) Access for all: housing design and the Disability Discrimination Act 1995, *Critical Social Policy*, 19, 3, 396–409.

Maglajlic, R., Brandon, D. and Given, D. (2000) Making direct payments a choice: a report on the research findings, *Disability and Society*, 15, 1, 99–114.

Magnusson, R.S. (2002) *Angels of Death: exploring the euthanasia underground*, New Haven, CT: Yale University Press.

Mann, T. (1967) Architectural barriers, *Caliper*, 24, 2, 8–9.

Mao, X. (1998) Chinese geneticists' views on ethical issues in genetic testing and screening: evidence for eugenics in China, *American Journal of Human Genetics*, 63, 3, 688–695.

Marfisi, C. (2002) Personally speaking: a critical reflection of factors which blur the original vision of personal assistance services, *Disability Studies Quarterly*, 22, 1, 25–30.

Marinelli, R.P. and Dell Orto, A.E. (1984) *The Psychological and Social Impact of Physical Disability*, New York: Springer Publishing.

Marquis, R. and Jackson, R. (2000) Quality of life and quality of service relationships: experiences of people with disabilities, *Disability and Society*, 15, 3, 411–426.

Marshall, T.H. (1950) *Citizenship and Social Class*, Cambridge: Cambridge University Press.

Martin, P. (1999) Genes and drugs: the social shaping of gene therapy and the reconstruction of genetic disease, in P. Conrad and J. Gabe (eds) *Sociological Perspectives on the New Genetics*, Oxford: Blackwell.

Martz, E. (2001) Acceptance of imperfection, *Disability Studies Quarterly*, 21, 3, 160–165.

Marwick, C. (2003) FDA halts gene therapy trials after leukaemia case in France, *British Medical Journal*, 326, 181, 25 January.

Meekosha, H. (2004) Drifting down the Gulf Stream: navigating the cultures of disability, *Disability and Society*, 19, 7, 721–734.

Meltzer, N., Singleton, A., Bebbington, P., Brugha, T. and Jenkins, R. (2002) *The Social and Economic Circumstances of Adults with Mental Disorders*, London: The Stationery Office.

Memmi, A. (1990) *The Coloniser and the Colonised*, London: Earthscan.

Mercer, G. (2002) Emancipatory research, in C. Barnes, M. Oliver and L. Barton (eds) *Disability Studies Today*, Cambridge: Polity.

Michailakis, D. (1997) When opportunity is the thing to be equalised, *Disability and Society*, 12, 1, 17–30.

Miller, L.L., Harvath, T.A., Ganzini, L., Goy, E.R., Delorit, M.A. and Jackson, A. (2004) Attitudes and experiences of Oregon hospice nurses and social workers regarding assisted suicide, *Palliative Medicine*, 18, 685–691.

Millet, K. (1971) *Sexual Politics*, New York: Avon Books.

Mohammed, M.A., Mant, J., Bentham, J., Stevens, A. and Hussain, S. (2005) Process of care and mortality of stroke patients with and without a do not resuscitate order in the West Midlands, UK, *International Journal for Quality in Health Care*, Advance Access, 7 October, 1–5.

Mohr, M. and Kettler, D. (1997) Ethical aspects of resuscitation, *British Journal of Anaesthesia*, 79: 253–259.

Moi, T. (1999) *What is a Woman?* Oxford: OUP.

Morgan, R., King, D., Prajapati, C. and Rowe, J. (1994) Views of elderly patients and their relatives on cardiopulmonary resuscitation, *British Medical Journal*, 308, 1677–1678.

Morris, J. (1991) *Pride Against Prejudice*, London: Women's Press.

Morris, J. (1992) Personal and political: a feminist perspective on researching physical disability, *Disability, Handicap and Society*, 7, 2, 157–166.

Morris, J. (1993a) *Independent Lives? Community care and disabled people*, London: Macmillan.

Morris, J. (1993b) Gender and disability, in J. Swain, V. Finkelstein, S. French and M. Oliver (eds) *Disabling Barriers, Enabling Environments*, London: Sage.

Morris, J. (1995) Creating a space for absent voices: disabled women's experience of receiving assistance with daily living activities, *Feminist Review*, 51, autumn, 68–93.

Morris, J. (ed.) (1996) *Encounters with Strangers: feminism and disability*, London: Women's Press.

Morris, J. (2004) Independent living and community care: a disempowering framework, *Disability and Society*, 19, 5, 427–442.

Mulvany, J. (2000) Disability, impairment or illness? The relevance of the social model of disability to the study of mental disorder, *Sociology of Health and Illness*, 22, 5, 582–601.

Murphy, D.J., Burrows, D., Santilli, S., Kemp, A.W., Tenner, S., Kelling, B. and Teno, S. (1994) The influence of the probability of survival on patients' preferences regarding CPR, *New England Journal of Medicine*, 330, 545–549.

Murray, P. (2002) *Hello! Are you listening? Disabled teenagers' experience of access to inclusive leisure*, York: Joseph Rowntree Foundation.

Newell, C. (1996) The disability rights movement in Australia: a note from the trenches, *Disability and Society*, 11, 3, 429–432.

Newell, C. (1998) Debates regarding governance: a disability perspective, *Disability and Society*, 13 , 2, 295–296.

Nirje, B. (1980) The normalization principle, in R. Flynn and K.E. Nitsch (eds) *Normalization, Social Integration and Community Services*, Baltimore, MD: University Park Press.

Noddings, N. (1984) *Caring: a feminine approach to ethics and moral education*, Berkeley, CA: University of California Press.

Nozick, R. (1975) *Anarchy, State and Utopia*, Oxford, Basil Blackwell.

Oakley, A. (1972) *Sex, Gender and Society*, London: Gower.

O'Brien, J. (1987) A guide to lifestyle planning: using the activities catalogue to integrate services and natural support systems, in B. Wilcox and G.T. Bellamy (eds) *The Activities Catalogue: an alternative curriculum for youth and adults with severe disabilities*, Baltimore, MD: Brookes.

O'Brien, R. (2001) *Crippled Justice: the history of modern disability policy in the workplace*, Chicago, IL: University of Chicago Press.

Oliver, M. (1983) *Social Work with Disabled People*, Basingstoke: Macmillan.

Oliver, M. (1989) Conductive education: if it wasn't so sad it would be funny, *Disability, Handicap and Society*, 4 , 2, 197–200.

Oliver, M. (1990) *The Politics of Disablement*, London: Macmillan.

Oliver, M. (1991) Speaking out: disabled people and state welfare, in G. Dalley (ed.) *Disability and Social Policy*, London: Policy Studies Institute.

Oliver, M. (1992a) Changing the social relations of research production? *Disability, Handicap and Society*, 7, 2, 101–114.

Oliver, M. (1992b) Intellectual masturbation: a rejoinder to Soder and Booth, *European Journal of Special Needs Education*, 7, 1, 20–28.

Oliver, M. (1993) *Disability, Citezenship and Empowerment*, Milton Keynes: Open University Press.

Oliver, M. (1996) *Understanding Disability: from theory to practice*, Basingstoke: Macmillan.

Oliver, M. (2004) The social model in action: if I had a hammer, in C. Barnes and G. Mercer (eds) *Implementing the Social Model of Disability: theory and research*, Leeds: The Disability Press.

Oliver, M. and Hasler, F. (1987) Disability and self-help: a case study of the Spinal Injuries Association, *Disability, Handicap and Society*, 2, 2, 113–125.

Oliver, M. and Zarb, G. (1989) The politics of disability: a new approach, *Disability, Handicap and Society*, 4, 3, 221–240.

Oliver, M. and Sapey, B. (1998) *Social Work with Disabled People* (second edition), Basingstoke: Palgrave Macmillan.

Orkin, S.H. and Motulsky, A.G. (1995) Report and recommendations of the panel to assess the NIH investment in research on gene therapy. Online. Available HTTP: <http://www.nih.gov/news/panelrep.html> (accessed 19 January).

Orr, R. (1999) The Gilgunn case: courage and questions, *Journal of Intensive Care Medicine*, 14, 1, 54–56.

Pahl, R. (2000) *On Friendship*, Cambridge: Polity.

*Paraplegia News* (1959) Kick him while he's down, Editorial *Paraplegia News*, 13, 132, 2.

Parens, E. (ed.) (2006) *Surgically Shaping Children*, Washington, DC: Georgetown University Press.

Parens, E. and Asch, A. (eds) (2000) *Prenatal Testing and Disability Rights*, Washington, DC: Georgetown University Press.

Parfit, D. (1984) *Reasons and Persons*, Oxford: Clarendon Press.

Paris, J.J., Cassem, E.H., Dec, G.W. and Reardon, F.E. (1999) Use of a DNR order over family objections: the case of Gilgunn v. MGH, *Journal of Intensive Care Medicine*, 14, 1, 41–45.

Paterson, K. and Hughes, B. (1999) Disability studies and phenomenology: the carnal politics of everyday life, *Disability and Society*, 14, 5, 597–610.

Paul, D.B. (1992) Eugenic anxieties, social realities, and political choices, *Social Research*, 59, 3, 663–683.

Payne, J., Brandon, D., Maglajlic, R. and Hawkes, A. (1998) *Direct Payments for Older People*, Cambridge: Anglia Polytechnic University.

Peace, S.M. (1998) Caring in place, in A. Brechin, J. Walmsley, J. Katz and S. Peace (eds) *Care Matters: concepts, practice and research in health and social care*, London: Sage.

Pearson, C. (2000) Money talks? Competing discourses in the implementation of direct payments, *Critical Social Policy*, 20, 4, 459–477.

Pearson, C. (2004) Keeping the cash under control: what's the problem with direct payments in Scotland? *Disability and Society*, 19, 1, 3–14.

Perske, T. (1988) *Circles of Friends*, Nashville, TN: Abingdon Press.

Pescosolido, B.A. (2001) The role of social networks in the lives of persons with disabilities, in G.L. Albrecht, K.D. Seelman and M. Bury (eds) *Handbook of Disability Studies*, Thousand Oaks: Sage.

Peters, S. (2000) Is there a disability culture? A syncretisation of three possible world views, *Disability and Society*, 15, 4, 583–601.

Pfeiffer, D. (1996) 'We won't go back': the ADA on the grass roots level, *Disability and Society*, 11, 2, 271–284.

Pfeiffer, D. (1998) The ICIDH and the need for its revision, *Disability and Society*, 3, 4, 503–523.

Pfeiffer, D. (2000) The devil is in the details: the ICIDH2 and the disability movement, *Disability and Society*, 15, 7, 1079–1082.

Pfeiffer, D. (2001) The conceptualization of disability, in S. Barnarrt and B.M. Altman (eds) *Exploring Theories and Expanding Methodologies: where are we and where do we need to go? Research in social science and disability volume 2*, Amsterdam: JAI.

Pinfold, V. (2004) *Social Participation*, report prepared for the Social Exclusion Unit, Rethink Severe Mental Illness.

Pitkeathley, J. (1989) *It's My Duty Isn't It? The plight of carers in our society*, London: Souvenir Press.

Prasad, R. (2003) Opportunity knock: campaigning charities fall short on jobs for disabled staff, *Guardian*, 12 March.

Press, N. and Browner, C. (1997) Why women say yes to prenatal diagnosis, *Social Science and Medicine*, 45, 979–989.

Price, D. and Barron, L. (1999) Developing independence: the experience of the Lawn-mowers Theatre Company, *Disability and Society*, 14, 6, 819–830.

Price, J. and Shildrick, M. (1998) Uncertain thoughts on the dis/abled body, in M. Shildrick and J. Price (eds) *Vital Signs: feminist reconfigurations of the biological body*, Edinburgh: Edinburgh University Press.

Priestley, M. (1998) Constructions and creations: idealism, materialism and disability theory, *Disability and Society*, 13, 1, 75–94.

Priestley, M. (2004) *Disability: a life course approach*, Cambridge: Polity.

Priestley, M., Corker, M. and Watson, N. (1999) Unfinished business: disabled children and disability identity, *Disability Studies Quarterly*, 19, 2, 87–98.

Race, D., Boxall, K. and Carson, I. (2005) Towards a dialogue for practice: reconciling social role valorisation and the social model of disability, *Disability and Society*, 20, 5, 507–521.

Rapp, R. (1997) *Testing Women, Testing the Fetus*, London: Routledge.

Rawles, S. (2004) Fringe benefits, *Guardian*, 31 March.

Rawls, J. (1972) *A Theory of Justice*, Oxford: Clarendon Press.

Read, J. (1998) Conductive education and the politics of disablement, *Disability and Society*, 13, 2, 279–293.

Reeve, D. (2003) 'Encounters with Strangers': Psycho-emotional dimensions of disability in everyday life, paper presented at the UK Disability Studies Conference, Lancaster. Online. Available HTTP: <http://www.disabilitystudies.net/index.php?content=23> (accessed 13 April 2006).

Reiskin, J. (1994) Suicide: political or personal? in B. Shaw (ed.) *The Ragged Edge*, Louisville KY: Avocado Press.

Resuscitation Council (2001) Decisions relating to cardiopulmonary resuscitation: a joint statement by the British Medical Association, the Resuscitation Council (UK) and the Royal College of Nursing. Online. Available HTTP: http://<www.resus.org.uk/pages/dnar.htm> (accessed 12 January 2006).

Reynolds, J. and Walmsley, J. (1998) Care, support or something else, in A. Brechin, J. Walmsley, J. Katz and S. Peace (eds) *Care Matters: concepts, practice and research in health and social care*, London: Sage.

Reynolds, T.M. (2003) Downs syndrome screening is unethical: views of today's research ethics committees, *Journal of Clinical Pathology*, 56, 268–270.

Rickell, A. (2003) Our disability is political, *Guardian*, 1 October.

Rickell, A. (2006) Key notes, *Disability Now*, 20 January.

Riddell, S., Pearson, C., Jolly, D., Barnes, D., Priestley, M. and Mercer, G. (2005) The development of direct payments in the UK: implications for social justice, *Social Policy and Society*, 4, 1, 75–85.

Riddick, B. (2000) An examination of the relationship between labelling and stigmatisation with special reference to dyslexia, *Disability and Society*, 15, 4, 653–668.

Ridley, J. and Jones, L. (2003) Direct what? The untapped potential of direct payments to mental health service users, *Disability and Society*, 18, 5, 643–658.

Riley, D. (1988) *Am I That Name?* Basingstoke: Macmillan.

Rioux, M. (1994) New research directions and paradigms: disability is not measles, in M. Rioux and M. Bach (eds) *Disability is not Measles: new research paradigms in disability*, North York: L'Institut Roeher Institute.

Rioux, M. and Bach, M. (eds) (1994) *Disability is not Measles: new research paradigms in disability*, North York: L'Institut Roeher Institute.

Robertson, J., Emerson, E., Gregory, N., Hatton, C., Kessissoglou, S., Hallam, A. and Linehan, C. (2001) Social networks of people with intellectual disabilities in residential settings, *Mental Retardation*, 39, 201–214.

Robson, P., Locke, M. and Dawson, J. (1997) *Consumerism or Democracy? User involvement in the control of voluntary organizations*, Bristol: The Policy Press.

Rock, P.J. (1996) Eugenics and euthanasia: a cause for concern for disabled people, particularly disabled women, *Disability and Society*, 11, 1, 121–128.

Rogers, L. (1999) Having disabled baby will be 'sin' says scientist, *Sunday Times*, 4 July.

Rose, P. and Kiger, G. (1995) Intergroup relations: political action and identity in the deaf community, *Disability and Society*, 10, 4, 521–528.

Russell, M. (2002) What disability civil rights cannot do: employment and political economy, *Disability and Society*, 17, 2, 117–135.

Safilios-Rothschild, C. (1970) *The Sociology and Social Psychology of Disability and Rehabilitation*, New York: Random House.

Safilios-Rothschild, C. (1976) Disabled persons' self-definitions and their implications for rehabilitation, in G.L. Albrecht (ed.) *The Sociology of Physical Disability and Rehabilitation*, Pittsburgh, PA: University of Pittsburgh Press.

Sample, I. (2005) Human stem cells allow paralysed mice to walk again, *Guardian*, 20 September.

Sapey, B., Stuart, J. and Donaldson, G. (2005) Increases in wheelchair use and perceptions of disablement, *Disability and Society*, 20, 5, 489–505.

Savulescu, J. (2001) Is current practice around late termination of pregnancy eugenic and discriminatory? Maternal interests and abortion, *Journal of Medical Ethics*, 27, 165–171.

Savulescu, J. (2002) Abortion, embryo destruction and the future of value argument, *Journal of Medical Ethics*, 28, 133–135.

Saxton, J. (1997) *What are charities for?* London: Third Sector Publishing.

Saxton, M. (2000) Why members of the disability community oppose prenatal diagnosis and selective abortion, in E. Parens and A. Asch (eds) *Prenatal Testing and Disability Rights*, Washington, DC: Georgetown University Press.

Sayers, G., Schofield, I. and Aziz, M. (1997) An analysis of CPR decision-making by elderly patients, *Journal of Medical Ethics*, 23, 207–212.

Scourfield, P. (2005) Implementing the Community Care (Direct Payments) Act: will the supply of personal assistants meet the demand and at what price? *Journal of Social Policy*, 34, 3, 469–488.

Scully, J.L. and Rehmann-Sutter, C. (2001) When norms normalize: the case of genetic 'enhancement', *Human Gene Therapy*, 12, 87–95.

Seale, C. (2006) National survey of end-of-life decisions made by UK medical practitioners, *Palliative Medicine*, 20, 1, 3–10.

Sevenhuijsen, S. (1998) *Citizenship and the Ethics of Care: feminist considerations on justice, morality and politics*, London: Routledge.

Seymour, W. and Lupton, D. (2004) Holding the line online: exploring wired relationships for people with disabilities, *Disability and Society*, 19, 4, 291–305.

Shakespeare, T. (1992) A response to Liz Crow, *Coalition*, September, 40–42.

Shakespeare, T. (1993) Disabled people's self-organisation: a new social movement? *Disability, Handicap and Society*, 8, 3, 249–264.

Shakespeare, T.W. (1994) Cultural representations of disabled people: dustbins for disavowal? *Disability and Society*, 9, 3, 283–299.

Shakespeare, T. (1995a) Back to the future? New genetics and disabled people, *Critical Social Policy*, 44, 45, 22–35.

Shakespeare, T. (1995b) Disability, identity, difference, in C. Barnes and G. Mercer (eds) *Chronic Illness and Disability: bridging the divide*, Leeds: Disability Press.

Shakespeare, T.W. (1998) Choices and rights: eugenics, genetics and disability equality, *Disability and Society*, 13, 5, 665–682.

Shakespeare, T.W. (1999a) Losing the plot? Discourses on genetics and disability, *Sociology of Health and Illness*, 21, 5, 669–688.

Shakespeare, T. (1999b) What is a disabled person? in M. Jones and L.B. Marks (eds) *Disability, Divers-ability and Legal Change*, The Hague: Martinus Nijhoff Publishers.

Shakespeare, T. (2000) *Help*, Birmingham: Venture Press.

Shakespeare, T.W. (2004) Social models of disability and other life strategies, *Scandinavian Journal of Disability Research*, 6, 1, 8–21.

Shakespeare, T.W. (2005a) The social context of reproductive choice, in D. Wasserman, J. Bickenbach and R. Wachbroit (eds) *Quality of Life and Human Difference: genetic testing, health care, and disability*, Cambridge: Cambridge University Press.

Shakespeare, T. (2005b) Disability, genetics and global justice, *Social Policy and Society*, 4, 1, 87–95.

Shakespeare, T.W. and Erickson, M. (2000) Different strokes: beyond biological essentialism and social constructionism, in S. Rose and H. Rose (eds) *Coming to life*, New York: Little, Brown.

Shakespeare, T.W. and Watson, N. (1995). Habeamus corpus? Disability studies and the issue of impairment, paper presented at Quincentennial Conference, University of Aberdeen.

Shakespeare, T.W. and Watson, N. (1997). Defending the social model, *Disability and Society*, 12, 2, 293–300.

Shakespeare, T. and Watson, N. (2001a) The social model of disability: an outdated ideology? in S. Barnarrt and B.M. Altman (eds). *Exploring Theories and Expanding Methodologies: where are we and where do we need to go?* Research in Social Science and Disability volume 2, Amsterdam: JAI.

Shakespeare, T. and Watson, N. (2001b) Making the difference: disability, politics and recognition, in G. Albrecht, K.D. Seelman and M. Bury (eds) *The Handbook of Disability Studies*, Thousand Oaks, CA: Sage.

Shakespeare, T., Gillespie-Sells, K. and Davies, D. (1996) *The Sexual Politics of Disability*, London: Cassell.

Sharp, K. and Earle, S. (2002) Feminism, abortion and disability: irreconcilable differences, *Disability and Society*, 17, 2, 137–146.

Shaw, B. (ed.) (1994) *The Ragged Edge*, Louisville KY: Avocado Press.

Shearer, A. (1981) A framework for independent living, in A. Walker with P. Townsend *Disability in Britain: a manifesto of rights*, Oxford: Martin Robertson.

Sheldon, S. and Wilkinson, S. (2001) Termination of pregnancy for reason of foetal disability: are there grounds for a special exception in law? *Medical Law Review*, 9, 85–109.

Sherry, M. (2002) 'If I only had a brain': examining the effects of brain injury in terms of disability, impairment, identity and embodiment, University of Queensland Ph.D. dissertation, unpublished.

Silvers, A. (1995) Reconciling equality to difference: caring (f)or justice for people with disabilities, *Hypatia*, 10, 1, 30–55.

Silvers, A. (1998) Protecting the innocents from physician assisted suicide, in M.P. Battin, Rhodes, R., Silvers, A. *Physician Assisted Suicide: expanding the debate*, London: Routledge.

Sim, A.J., Milner, J., Love, J. and Lishman, J. (1998) Definitions of need: can disabled people and care professionals agree? *Disability and Society*, 13, 1, 53–74.

Singer, J. (1999) 'Why can't you be normal for once in your life?' From a 'problem with no name' to the emergence of a new category of difference, in M. Corker and S. French, *Disability Discourse*, Buckingham: Open University Press.

Singer, P. (1993) *Practical Ethics*, New York: Cambridge University Press.

Skär, L. and Tam, M. (2001) My assistant and I: disabled children's and adolescents' roles and relationships to their assistants, *Disability and Society*, 16, 7, 917–932.

Skär, R.N.L. (2003) Peer and adult relationships of adolescents with disabilities, *Journal of Adolescence*, 26, 635–649.

Smart, A. (2003) Reporting the dawn of the post-genomic era: who wants to live forever? *Sociology of Health and Illness*, 25, 1, 24–49.

Smith, A. and Twomey, B (2002) Labour market experience of people with disabilities, *Labour Market Trends*, August, 415–427.

Smith, B. and Sparkes, A.C. (2004) Men, sport and spinal cord injury: an analysis of metaphors and narrative types, *Disability and Society*, 19, 6, 613–626.

Smith, N., Middleton, S., Ashton-Brooks, K., Cox, L. and Dobson, B. with Reith, L. (2005) *Disabled People's Costs of Living: 'more than you would think'*, York: Joseph Rowntree Foundation.

Smittkamp, J. (1964) 'NPF Director's Report', *Paraplegia News*, 17, 185, 6.

Sobsey, R. (1994) An illusion of autonomy: questioning physician-assisted suicide and euthanasia. Brief submitted to the Special Senate Committee on Euthanasia and Assisted Suicide, Canada: Winnipeg: University of Alberta Developmental Disabilities Centre.

Söder, M. (1989) Disability as a social construct: the labelling approach revisited, *European Journal of Special Needs Education*, 4, 2, 117–129.

Spandler, H. (2004) Friend or foe? Towards a critical assessment of direct payments, *Critical Social Policy*, 79, 24 (2), 187–209.

Spriggs, M. and Savulescu, J. (2002) The Perruche judgement and the 'right not to be born', *Journal of Medical Ethics*, 28, 63–64.

Stacey, C.L. (2005) Finding dignity in dirty work: the constraints and rewards of low-wage home care labour, *Sociology of Health and Illness*, 27, 6, 831–854.

Stainton, T. and Boyce, S. (2004) I have got my life back: users' experiences of direct payments, *Disability and Society*, 19, 5, 443–454.

Stalker, K., Baron S., Riddell S. and Wilkinson, H. (1999) Models of disability: the relationship between theory and practice in non-statutory organisations, *Critical Social Policy*, 19, 1, 5–29.

Statham, H. and Solomou, W. (2001) *When a Baby has an Abnormality: a study of parents' experiences*, Cambridge: Centre for Family Research.

Stark, S. (2001) Creating disability in the home: the role of environmental barriers in the United States, *Disability and Society*, 16, 1, 37–50.

St Claire, L. (1986) Mental retardation: impairment or handicap? *Disability, Handicap and Society*, 1, 3, 233–243.

Stevens, A. (2004) Closer to home: a critique of British government policy towards accomodating learning disabled people in their own homes, *Critical Social Policy*, 79, 24 (2), 233–254.

Stewart, K., Spice, C. and Rai, G.S. (2003) Where now with Do Not Attempt Resuscitation decisions? *Age and Ageing*, 32, 143–148.

Stockdale, A. (1999) Waiting for the cure: mapping the social relations of human gene therapy research, in P. Conrad and J. Gabe (eds) *Sociological Perspectives on the New Genetics*, Oxford: Blackwell.

Stone, D.A. (1985) *The Disabled State*, Basingstoke: Macmillan.

Stone, E. (1997) From the research notes of a foreign devil: disability research in China, in C. Barnes and G. Mercer (eds) *Doing Disability Research*, Leeds: The Disability Press.

Stone, E. (1999) Modern slogan, ancient script: impairment and disability in the Chinese language, in M. Corker and S. French, *Disability Discourse*, London: Sage.

Stone, S.D. (1995) The myth of bodily perfection, *Disability and Society*, 10, 4, 413–424.

Stortingsmelding 88 (1966–67) *Om utviklingen av omsorgen for funksjonshemmede* (Concerning the development of social care services for the disabled), Oslo: Ministry of Social Affairs.

Sutherland, A. (1981) *Disabled we stand*, London: Souvenir Press.

Swain, J. and French, S. (2000) Towards an affirmation model of disability, *Disability and Society*, 15, 4, 569–582.

Swain, J., French, S. and Cameron, C. (eds) (2003) *Controversial Issues in a Disabling Society*, Buckingham: Open University Press.

Swain, J., French, S., Barnes, C. and Thomas, C. (eds) (2004) *Disabling Barriers – Enabling Environments*, London: Sage.

Szasz, T. (1974) *The Myth of Mental Illness: foundations of a theory of personal conduct*, New York: Harper and Row.

Tajfel, H. (1978) *The Social Psychology of Minorities*, London: Minority Rights Group.

Taylor, M. (1997) *The Best of Both Worlds: the voluntary sector and local government*, York: Joseph Rowntree Foundation.

Taylor, S.J. and Bogdan, R. (1989) On accepting relationships between people with mental retardation and non-disabled people: towards an understanding of acceptance, *Disability, Handicap and Society*, 4, 1, 21–36.

Thomas, C. (1998) The body and society: impairment and disability, paper presented at BSA Annual Conference *Making Sense of the Body*, Edinburgh.

Thomas, C. (1999) *Female forms: experiencing and understanding disability*, Buckingham: Open University Press.

Thomas, C. (2004a) How is disability understood? *Disability and Society*, 19, 6, 563–568.

Thomas, C. (2004b) Rescuing a social relational understanding of disability, *Scandinavian Journal of Disability Research*, 6, 1, 22–36.

Thomas, D. (1982) *The Experience of Handicap*, London: Methuen.

Tiefer, L. (1995) *Sex is Not a Natural Act*, Boulder, CO: Westview Press.

Tierney, S. (2001) A reluctance to be defined 'disabled': how can the social model of disability enhance understanding of anorexia? *Disability and Society*, 16, 5, 749–764.

Timpanaro, S. (1975) *On Materialism*, London: New Left Books.

Topliss, E. (1979) *Provision for the Disabled*, Oxford: Blackwell.

Topliss, E. (1982) *Social Responses to Handicap*, Harlow: Longman.

Tøssebro, J. (2004) Understanding disability, *Scandinavian Journal of Disability Research*, 6, 1, 3–7.

Tøssebro, J. and Kittelsaa, A. (2004) Studying the living conditions of disabled people: approaches and problems, in J. Tøssebro and A. Kittelsaa (eds) *Exploring the Living Conditions of Disabled People*, Lund: Studentlitteratur.

Townsend, P. (1981) Elderly people with disabilities, in A. Walker with P. Townsend, *Disability in Britain: a manifesto of rights*, Oxford: Martin Robertson.

Traustadóttir, R. (1993) The gendered context of friendships, in A.N. Amado (ed.) *Friendship and Community Connections between People with and without Developmental Disabilities*, Baltimore, MD: Paul Brookes Publishing.

Traustadóttir, R. (2000) Friendship: love or work? in R. Traustadóttir and K. Johnson (eds) *Women with Intellectual Disabilities: finding a place in the world*, London: Jessica Kingsley Publishers.

Traustadóttir, R. (2001) Research with others: reflections on representation, difference and othering, *Scandinavian Journal of Disability Research*, 3, 2, 9–28.

Tregaskis, C. (2004a) *Constructions of Disability: researching the interface between disabled and non-disabled people*, London: Routledge.

Tregaskis, C. (2004b) Applying the social model in practice: some lessons from countryside recreation, *Disability and Society* 19, 6, 601–612.

Tremain, S. (1998) Feminist approaches to naturalizing disabled bodies or, does the social model of disablement rest upon a mistake? Paper presented at Annual Meeting of the Society for Disability Studies, Oakland, CA.

Tremain, S. (2002) On the subject of impairment, in M. Corker and T. Shakespeare (eds) *Disability/Postmodernity: embodying disability theory*, London: Continuum.

Tremblay, M., Campbell, A. and Hudson, G.L. (2005) When elevators were for pianos: an oral history account of the civilian experience of using wheelchairs in Canadian society. The first twenty-five years: 1945–1970, *Disability and Society*, 20, 2, 103–116.

Tronto, J.C. (1993) *Moral Boundaries: a political argument for an ethic of care*, London: Routledge.

Tucker, B.P. (1998) Deaf culture, cochlear implants, and elective disability, *Hastings Center Report*, 28, 4, 6–14.

Turner, B.S. (2001) Disability and the sociology of the body, in G.L. Albrecht, K.D. Seelman and M. Bury (eds) *The Handbook of Disability Studies*, Thousand Oaks, CA: Sage.

Ungerson, C. (1987) *Policy is Personal: sex gender and informal care*, London: Tavistock.

United Nations (2003) *The Standard Rules on the Equalization of Opportunities for Persons with Disabilities*, New York: United Nations.

UPIAS (1976) *Fundamental Principles of Disability*, London: UPIAS.

Ursic, C. (1996) Social (and disability) policy in the new democracies of Europe (Slovenia by way of example), *Disability and Society*, 11, 1, 91–105.

Van den Ven, L., Post, M., de Witte, L. and van den Heuvel, W. (2005) It takes two to tango: the integration of people with disabilities into society, *Disability and Society*, 20, 3, 311–329.

Van der Klift, E. and Kunc, N. (1994) Hell-bent on helping: benevolence, friendship and the politics of help. Online. Available HTTP: <www.noormemma.com/arhellbe.htm> (accessed 2 September 2004).

Vanier, J. (1999) *Becoming Human*, London: Darton, Longman and Todd.

Vehmas, S. (2002) Parental responsibility and the morality of selective abortion, *Ethical Theory and Moral Practice*, 5, 463–484.

Vehmas, S. (2003a) Live and let die? Disability in bioethics, *New Review of Bioethics*, 1, 1, 145–157.

Vehmas, S. (2003b) The grounds for preventing impairments: a critique, in M. Härry and T. Takala (eds) *Scratching the Surface of Bioethics*, New York/Amsterdam: Rodopi.

Vehmas, S. (2004) Ethical analysis of the concept of disability, *Mental Retardation*, 42, 3, 209–222.

Vehmas, S. (2006) The who or what of Steve: severe cognitive impairment and its implications, *Scandinavian Journal of Disability Research*, forthcoming.

Vernon, A. (1996) A stranger in many camps: the experience of disabled black and ethnic minority women, in J. Morris (ed.) *Encounters with Strangers: feminism and disability*, London: Women's Press.

Vernon, A. (1999) The dialectics of multiple identities and the disabled people's movement, *Disability and Society*, 14, 3, 385–398.

Vernon, A. and Qureshi, H. (2000) Community care and independence: self-sufficiency or empowerment? *Critical Social Policy*, 63, 20 (2), 255–276.

Voet, R. (1998) *Feminism and Citizenship*, London: Sage.

Wagg, A., Kinrions, M. and Stewart, K. (1995) Cardiopulmonary resuscitation: doctors and nurses expect too much, *Journal of the Royal College of Physicians of London*, 29, 20–24.

Walker, A. with Townsend, P. (1981) *Disability in Britain: a manifesto of rights*, Oxford: Martin Robertson.

Wall, P. (1999) *Pain: the science of suffering*, London: Weidenfeld and Nicholson.

Walmsley, J. (2001) Normalisation, emancipatory research and inclusive research, *Disability and Society*, 16, 2, 187–205.

Warren, M.A. (1993) Abortion, in P. Singer (ed.) *A Companion to Ethics*, Oxford: Blackwell.

Warren, M.A. (1997) *Moral Status: obligations to persons and other living things*, Oxford: Clarendon Press.

Wasserman, D. (2001) Philosophical issues in the definition and social response to disability, in G. Albrecht, K. Seelman and M. Bury (eds) *The Handbook of Disability Studies*, Thousand Oaks, CA: Sage.

Watson, N. (2002) Well, I know this is going to sound very strange to you, but I don't see myself as a disabled person: identity and disability, *Disability and Society*, 17, 5, 509–527.

Watson, N (2003) Daily denials: the routinisation of oppression and resistance, in N. Watson and S. Riddell (eds) *Disability, Culture and Identity*, Harlow: Pearson Education.

Watson, N., McKie, L., Hughes, B., Hopkins, D. and Gregory, S. (2004) (Inter)dependence, needs and care: the potential for disability and feminist theorists to develop an emancipatory model, *Sociology*, 38, 2, 331–350.

Weeks, J., Heaphy, B. and Donovan, C. (2001) *Same Sex Intimacies: families of choice and other life experiments*, London: Routledge.

Wendell, S. (1996) *The Rejected Body: feminist philosophical reflections on disability*, New York: Routledge.

Wertz, D. (1998) Eugenics is alive and well, *Science in Context*, 11, 3 & 4, 493–510.

White-van Mourik, M. (1994) Termination of a second-trimester pregnancy for fetal abnormality: psychosocial aspects, in A. Clarke (ed.) *Genetic Counselling: practice and principles*, London: Routledge.

Wikler, D. (1999) Can we learn from eugenics? *Journal of Medical Ethics*, 25, 2 183–194.

Williams, C., Alderson, P. and Farsides, B. (2002) What constitutes 'balanced' information in the practitioners' portrayals of Down's syndrome? *Midwifery*, 18, 230–237.

Williams, C., Kitzinger, J. and Henderson, L. (2003) Envisaging the embryo in stem cell research: rhetorical strategies and media reporting of the ethical debates, *Sociology of Health and Illness*, 25, 7, 793–814.

Williams, C., Sandall, J., Lewando-Hundt, G., Heyman, B., Spencer, K. and Grellier, R. (2005) Women as moral pioneers? Experiences of first trimester antenatal screening, *Social Science and Medicine*, 61, 1983–1992.

Williams, F. (2001) In and beyond New Labour: towards a new political ethics of care, *Critical Social Policy*, 21, 4, 467–493.

Williams, G. (1983) The movement for independent living: an evaluation and a critique, *Social Science and Medicine*, 17, 15, 1003–1010.

Williams, I. (1989) *The Alms Trade: Charities, past, present and future*, London: Unwin Hyman.

Williams, S.J. (1999) Is anybody there? Critical realism, chronic illness and the disability debate, *Sociology of Health and Illness*, 21, 6, 797–819.

Wilson, A., Riddell, S., Baron, S. (2000) Welfare for those who can? The impact of the quasi-market on the lives of people with learning difficulties, *Critical Social Policy*, 20, 4, 479–502.

Wolfensburger, W. (1972) *The Principle of Normalisation in Human Services*, Toronto: National Institue on Mental Retardation.

Wolfensburger, W. (1989) Human service policies: the rhetoric versus the reality, in L. Barton (ed.) *Disability and Dependency*, Lewes: Falmer Press.

Wood, R. (1991) Care of disabled people, in G. Dalley (ed.) *Disability and Social Policy*, London: Policy Studies Institute.

Wood Mak, Y.Y. and Elwyn, G. (2005) Voices of the terminally ill: uncovering the meaning of desire for euthanasia, *Palliative Medicine*, 19, 343–350.

Woods, S. (2002) Respect for autonomy and palliative care, in H. Ten Have and D. Clark (eds) *The Ethics of Palliative Care*, Buckingham: Open University Press.

Woods, S. (2005) Respect for persons: autonomy and palliative care, *Medicine Health Care and Philosophy*, 8, 243–253.

World Health Organization (1980) *International Classification of Impairments, Disabilities and Handicaps*, Geneva: World Health Organization.

Wright, B.A. (1960) *Physical disability: a psychological approach*, New York: Harper and Row.

Wuthnow, R. (1991) *Acts of Compassion: caring for others and helping ourselves*, Princeton, NJ: Princeton University Press.

Yamaki, C.K. and Yamazaki, Y. (2004) 'Instruments', 'employees', 'companions', 'social assets': understanding relationships between persons with disabilities and their assistants in Japan, *Disability and Society*, 19, 1, 31–46.

Young, D.A. and Quibell, R. (2000) Why rights are never enough: rights, intellectual disability and understanding, *Disability and Society*, 15, 5, 747–764.

Young, I.M. (1990) *Justice and The Politics of Difference*, Princeton, NJ: Princeton University Press.

Young, I.M. (1997) Asymmetrical reciprocity: on moral respect, wonder, and enlarged thought, *Constellations*, 3, 3, 340–363.

Zarb, G. (1997) Researching disabling barriers, in C. Barnes and G. Mercer (eds) *Doing Disability Research*, Leeds: The Disability Press.

Zarb, G. and Nadash, P. (1995) *Direct Payments for Personal Assistance*, Social Policy Research Findings No. 64, London: Policy Studies Institute.

Zeiler, K. (2005) *Chosen Children? An empirical study and a philosophical analysis of moral aspects of pre-implantation genetic diagnosis and germ-line gene therapy*, Linköping: Linköping University Studies in Art and Science.

Zola, I. (1983) *Socio-medical Inquiries: recollections, reflections and reconsiderations*, Philadelphia, PA: Temple University Press.

Zola, I.K. (1977) Healthism and disabling medicalisation, in I. Illich (ed.) *Disabling Professions*, London: Marion Boyars.

Zola, I.K. (1989) Towards the necessary universalizing of a disability policy, *The Milbank Quarterly*, 67 (2), 2, 401–428.

Zola, I.K. (1994) Towards inclusion: the role of people with disabilities in policy and research issues in the United States – a historical and political analysis, in M. Rioux and M. Bach (eds) (1994) *Disability is not Measles: new research paradigms in disability*, North York: L'Institut Roeher Institute.

Zuczewski, M.G. (2001) Disability: an agenda for bioethics, *American Journal of Bioethics*, 1, 3, 36–44.

# Index